Student Workbook for

Darby and Walsh Dental Hygiene: Theory and Practice

Sixth Edition

Margaret Lemaster, MS, BSDH, RDH
Adjunct Professor
School of Dentistry
Virginia Commonwealth University
Richmond, VA

ELSEVIER

Elsevier
3251 Riverport Lane
St. Louis, Missouri 63043

STUDENT WORKBOOK FOR DARBY AND WALSH DENTAL HYGIENE: ISBN: 978-0-323-88274-3
THEORY AND PRACTICE, SIXTH EDITION

Notice

Practitioners and researchers must always rely on their own experience and knowledge in evaluating and using any information, methods, compounds or experiments described herein. Because of rapid advances in the medical sciences, in particular, independent verification of diagnoses and drug dosages should be made. To the fullest extent of the law, no responsibility is assumed by Elsevier, authors, editors or contributors for any injury and/or damage to persons or property as a matter of products liability, negligence or otherwise, or from any use or operation of any methods, products, instructions, or ideas contained in the material herein.

Previous edition copyrighted 2020

Senior Content Strategist: Kelly Skelton
Senior Content Development Specialist: Kathleen Nahm
Publishing Services Manager: Deepthi Unni
Senior Project Manager: Kamatchi Madhavan
Design Direction: Gopal Venkatraman

Printed in India

Last digit is the print number: 9   8   7   6   5   4   3   2   1

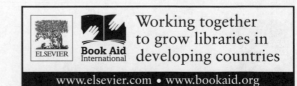

To the next generation of students – make us proud!

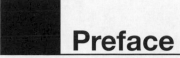

Preface

Student Workbook for Darby and Walsh Dental Hygiene: Theory and Practice, 6th Edition, is the essential review, practice, and application resource to reinforce the concepts and skills presented in *Darby and Walsh Dental Hygiene: Theory and Practice,* the comprehensive and evidence-based core text used to train dental hygiene students from day 1 through graduation and beyond. Student Workbook chapters correlate to textbook chapters and provide ample review questions and exercises, competency skills evaluation sheets, case studies with questions, and information for the clinical practice and professional portfolio. Applicable chapters contain a review of video procedures located on the textbook's companion website. This workbook is the essential practice and review needed to ensure didactic and clinical success!

KEY FEATURES

1. Correlation with textbook chapters
2. Practice and review questions
3. Competency skill checklists
4. Patient case studies
5. Video review sections
6. Professional portfolio exercises
7. Perforated pages

STUDENT WORKBOOK CONTENT OVERVIEW

Chapter Competencies: Each chapter begins with objectives/competencies outlined in the textbook chapter.

General Instructions: Each section of the workbook includes brief instructions for students. These instructions explain the procedure for answering each question. The instructions appear below each section title and are italicized.

Vocabulary Exercises: These exercises are fill-in-the-blank or multiple-choice formats and cover key terms in the corresponding textbook chapter. The key terms are not listed in the textbook but are bolded throughout the chapters.

Competency Skills Checklists: Each procedure in the textbook has a corresponding Competency Checklist in the workbook. The Competency Checklist grading rubrics are in table format and include self, peer, and instructor evaluation space and performance criteria listing steps.

Practice and Review Questions: Questions span three cognitive levels: recall, comprehension, and application. All questions reflect information within the corresponding textbook chapter. The questions are organized by type:

   Short Answer Questions are open-ended questions that can be answered based on the information in the corresponding textbook chapter.
   Fill in the Blank Statements include questions with words and/or phrases that can be answered based on the information in the corresponding textbook chapter.
   Multiple-Choice Questions include question a stem and four answer choices (A-D) with one correct answer.
   Case Study scenarios are presented for each chapter with accompanying critical thinking questions.
   Video review questions are provided for several textbook chapters, referred to as "Dental Hygiene Procedure Videos," and will be accessible through Evolve.

Professional Portfolio Guide includes exercises and recommendations for students to create a professional portfolio.

ANSWERS

All answers will be posted on Evolve in the Instructor resources.

Contents

The Dental Hygiene Profession

COMPETENCIES

1. Apply knowledge of the discipline of dental hygiene, the dental hygienist, and the dental hygiene process of care to succinctly elucidate the primary focus of dental hygiene and approaches taken by dental hygienists to prevent oral diseases and foster overall wellness.
2. Relate the concepts in the metaparadigm for the discipline of dental hygiene to differences in clients, environment.
3. Consider the professional roles of the dental hygienist to determine if more than one of them might appeal to you, and why.
4. Compare and contrast the different workforce models for dental hygienists and how they are impacted by professional regulation in the US and Canada.
5. Contemplate the role and importance of various professional dental hygiene associations, highlight why participation is important for professionals, and select at least two of interest.

SHORT ANSWER QUESTIONS

1. List the six steps of the Dental Hygiene Process of Care

2. List and briefly describe the four paradigm concepts of dental hygiene.

3. List the four main professional associations that represent dental hygiene.

_____

_____

_____

_____

_____

_____

_____

_____

4. List the seven roles of the professional dental hygienist

_____

_____

_____

_____

_____

_____

_____

_____

_____

_____

_____

_____

5. List and briefly describe the various dental hygiene workforce models.

_____

_____

_____

_____

_____

_____

6. List common elements in dental and dental hygiene practice acts in states and provinces that regulate the practice of dental hygiene.

FILL IN THE BLANK STATEMENTS

Select the best term from the chapter and complete the following statements.

1. _____ is the art and science of preventive oral health care, including the management of behaviors to prevent oral disease and to promote health.

2. _____ is the primary oral health care professionals that are licensed and have graduated from accredited dental hygiene programs in institutions of higher education.

3. _____ is the foundation of professional dental hygiene practice and provides a framework for delivering high-quality dental hygiene care to all types of clients in any environment or professional role.

4. _____ is the collection and analysis of oral health data collected through a systematic, comprehensive individualized assessment of the client (individual/patient, group, community, population) who may be with or at risk for oral disease or complications.

5. _____ involves identifying an individual's health behaviors, attitudes, and oral health care needs within the scope of services the dental hygienist is licensed and educated to provide.

6. _____ phase of care is to select, prioritize, and sequence dental hygiene interventions for realistic, overall patient goals to move the patient toward oral health.

7. _____ is the process of completing the plan and engaging the patient as an active participant in their personalized care.

8. _____ is feedback on effectiveness of oral and health conditions and patient behaviors by collecting and interpreting data using measurable outcomes.

9. _____ is accurately recording all assessment findings, treatment planned and delivered, patient communication, treatment outcomes, and recommendations.

10. _____ is the ability of a dental hygienist to initiate treatment based on their assessment of a patient's needs without the specific authorization of a dentist, treat the patient without the presence of a dentist, and maintain a provider-patient relationship.

11. _____ is dentists and dental hygienists working together as colleagues, each offering professional expertise for the goal of providing optimum oral health care to the public.

12. _____ is shared responsibility and collaboration among health care professionals in patient-centered care health care delivery systems to attain optimal health outcomes.

MULTIPLE CHOICE QUESTIONS

Complete each question by circling the best answer.

1. Which licensed dental hygienist and graduate from an accredited dental hygiene program is a primary oral health care provider of dental hygiene services directly to patients and has an expanded scope of care?
   a. Public health dental hygienist
   b. Expanded function dental hygienist
   c. General supervision practitioner
   d. Mid-level oral health practitioner

2. The Dental Hygiene Practice Act includes all of the following elements EXCEPT:
   a. Establishes criteria for dental hygiene education, licensure, and relicensure
   b. Defines the legal scope of dental hygiene practice
   c. Protects the public by making illegal the practice of dental assisting by uncredentialled and unlicensed persons
   d. Creates a board empowered with legal authority to oversee the policies and procedures affecting the dental hygiene practice in that jurisdiction

3. Which stage of the dental hygiene process of care includes completing a thorough medical history on a patient?
   a. Assessment
   b. Dental hygiene diagnosis
   c. Planning
   d. Implementation

4. Mid-Level Oral Health Care Workforce Models outcomes should reflect all of the following concepts EXCEPT:
   a. Quality dental care
   b. Primary dental care
   c. Inexpensive dental insurance
   d. Overall improved collective health

5. Which stage of the dental hygiene process of care includes collaborating with a patient and developing realistic goals?
   a. Assessment
   b. Dental hygiene diagnosis
   c. Planning
   d. Implementation

6. A practitioner who owns their own business, or independent practice, and provides preventive oral health care services to the public as a primary care provider where permitted by law is considered:
   a. Interprofessional dental hygienist
   b. Independent practitioner
   c. Advanced practice dental hygienist
   d. Dental therapist

7. A formal, voluntary process that establishes a minimum set of national standards that promote and ensure quality across educational institutions and programs and serves as a mechanism to protect the public is:
   a. Licensure
   b. Professional regulation
   c. Dental Hygiene Practice Act
   d. Accreditation

8. Which stage of the dental hygiene process of care includes recording and detailing assessment findings, treatment planned and delivered, patient communication, treatment outcomes, and recommendations?
   a. Assessment
   b. Dental hygiene diagnosis
   c. Planning
   d. Implementation
   e. Documentation

CASE STUDY

You are a recent graduate from an accredited dental hygiene school. Although you had originally planned on employment in a private practice setting, you are intrigued by the public health setting. What steps do you take to investigate the public health setting? Who would you contact?

2 Dental Hygiene Metaparadigm Concepts and Conceptual Models Applied to Practice

COMPETENCIES

1. Discuss the dental hygiene metaparadigm and its four paradigm concepts.
2. Define conceptual model.
3. Discuss the key features of the Dental Hygiene Human Needs Model, illustrate how the model enables the dental hygienist to diagnose patient needs based on assessment and/or formulate a plan of action to help meet the need, and apply the model to two fictional patient cases.
4. Discuss the key features and domains of the Oral Health-Related Quality of Life Model, illustrate how the model enables the dental hygienist to diagnose patient needs based on assessment and/or formulate a plan of action to help meet the need, and apply the model to two fictional patient cases.
5. Discuss the key features and domains of the Client Self-Care Commitment Model, illustrate how the model enables the dental hygienist to diagnose patient needs based on assessment and/or formulate a plan of action to help meet the need, and apply the model to two fictional patient cases.

SHORT ANSWER QUESTIONS

1. What are the four dental hygiene concepts from a clinical practice perspective?

_____

_____

_____

_____

_____

_____

_____

_____

2. List the eight Human Needs Conceptual Model deficits.

_____

_____

_____

_____

_____

_____

_____

_____

_____

_____

_____

3. What are the six key elements of the Oral Health-Related Quality of Life Model?

_____

_____

_____

_____

_____

_____

4. What are the domains of the Client Self-Care Commitment Model?

_____

_____

_____

_____

_____

_____

_____

FILL IN THE BLANK STATEMENTS

Select the best term from the chapter and complete the following statements.

1. _____ is a distinct set of concepts or thought patterns, including theories, and standards that influence how we view different situations.

2. _____ is a more general statement of a discipline and functions as a framework in which the more restricted structures of conceptual models develop.

3. _____ is a term that identifies the recipient of dental hygiene actions who may be an individual, a community, or a particular group.

4. _____ is the surroundings in which the client and dental hygienist interact.

5. _____ is the client's state of well-being on a continuum from maximum wellness to maximum illness.

6. _____ are the interventions provided by a dental hygienist to promote oral wellness and wellness and prevent oral disease.

7. _____ is composed of ideas and the theoretical linkages between them, which together describe a particular relationship.

8. _____ is a multidimensional concept that includes a subjective evaluation of the individual's oral health, functional well-being, emotional well-being, expectations of and satisfaction with care, and sense of self.

9. _____ proposes that the relationships among the domains and the interaction between the client and the dental hygienist can empower clients to make decisions that will enhance their own health through commitment and compliance.

10. _____ enables, mediates, and advocates for client-centered human need fulfilment and allows dental hygienists to provide a holistic and humanistic perspective for dental hygiene care.

MULTIPLE CHOICE QUESTIONS

Complete each question by circling the best answer.

1. Your 20-year-old female patient presents with rampant caries. The Human Needs Conceptual model deficit is:
   a. Freedom from Pain
   b. Skin and Mucous Membrane Integrity of the Head and Neck
   c. Biologically Sound and Functional Dentition
   d. Conceptualization and Problem Solving

2. Your 55-year-old patient has high blood pressure and uncontrolled type 2 diabetes. The Human Needs Conceptual model deficit is:
   a. Protection from Health Risks
   b. Freedom from Fear and Stress
   c. Conceptualization and Problem Solving
   d. Responsibility for Oral Health

3. Your 35-year-old patient reports that he has nocturnal bruxism. The Human Needs Conceptual model deficit is:
   a. Protection from Health Risks
   b. Freedom from Pain
   c. Skin and Mucous Membrane Integrity of the Head and Neck
   d. Biologically Sound and Functional Dentition

4. When setting priorities for unmet human needs, which of the following deficits should be treated FIRST?
   a. Necrotizing Ulcerative Periodontitis: Skin and Mucous Membrane Integrity of the Head and Neck
   b. No dental exam in 3 years: Responsibility for Oral Health
   c. Patient views fluoride as a toxin and refuses fluoride treatment: Protection from Health Risks
   d. Patient is getting married soon and wants teeth whitened as soon as possible: Wholesome Facial Image

5. All of the following domains are components if the Client Self-Care Commitment Model EXCEPT:
   a. Assessment Domain
   b. Commitment Domain
   c. Evaluation Domain
   d. Planning Domain

6. The Oral Health-Related Quality of Life Model emphasizes respecting a patient's individuality as important to help patients achieve their desired health outcomes. This person-centered model allows the dental hygienist to learn from the patient about their needs, and the patient learns from the dental hygienist about oral/systemic health.
   a. Both statements are true.
   b. Both statements are false.
   c. The first statement is true and the second statement is false.
   d. The first statement is false and the second statement is true.

7. Dental hygienists help individuals, families, groups, and communities prevent oral disease and provide interventions and programs specifically designed to foster oral and general health. This statement reflects which The Oral Health-Related Quality of Life Model domain?
   a. Health and Preclinical Disease Domain
   b. Functional Status Domain
   c. Health Perceptions Domain
   d. General Quality of Life Domain

8. Your 60-year-old female patient is recovering from a stroke. Her speech is affected, and she is currently in speech therapy twice a week. Which domain of the Oral Health-Related Quality of Life Model does this address?
   a. Biological and Physical Clinical Variables
   b. Symptom Status Domain
   c. Functional Status Domain
   d. General Quality of Life Domain

9. The Client Self-Care Commitment Model uses components of all of the following models EXCEPT:
   a. Dental Hygiene Human Needs Model
   b. Client Empowerment Model
   c. Explanatory Model
   d. Oral Health-Related Quality of Life Model

10. The process of dental hygiene care requires ethical, comprehensive care using best practices supported by evidence. The best conceptual model that exists for private practice is the Human Needs Conceptual Model.
    a. Both statements are true.
    b. Both statements are false.
    c. The first statement is true and the second statement is false.
    d. The first statement is false and the second statement is true.

Chapter 2 **Dental Hygiene Metaparadigm Concepts and Conceptual Models Applied to Practice**

CASE STUDY: MRS. GRAHAM

Mrs. Graham is a 78-year-old retired high school teacher who presents for her 4-month periodontal maintenance appointment. Health history findings include normal vital signs, history of hypertension, seasonal allergies, and asthma. She reports compliance with anti-hypertensive and bronchodilation medications. She sees her primary care physician regularly. She is active with her church and is an avid bird watcher. She walks several times a week and occasionally swims at the local YMCA.

Mrs. Graham uses a manual toothbrush and fluoridated toothpaste twice a day, interdental picks twice a week. She drinks two colas a day and two cups of sweetened coffee each morning. She admits to eating more candy than she should.

Using the data from this patient, develop a Human Needs Conceptual model for treatment.

Age	78	SCENARIO
Gender	F	**EOE/IOE:**
Height	5'4"	Xerostomia
Weight	140 lb	Coated tongue
B/P	140/85 mm Hg	Localized slight subgingival calculus
Chief Complaint		Moderate supragingival calculus on the lingual of mandibular anterior teeth
Medical History	Hypertension Asthma – controlled Arthritis	Generalized marginal and interproximal biofilm **Periodontal Findings:** Chronic localized periodontitis in the posterior
Current Medications	Hydrochlorothizide Singular Advair Proventil	3-5 mm probing depths 4-6 mm clinical attachment loss Bleeding upon probing Class I furcation on all first molars
Social History	Non-drinker Non-smoker	**Radiographic Findings:** Horizontal bone loss **Dental Findings:** Numerous crowns and restorations Root caries on teeth #3, 4, 11, 12, 14

Dental Hygiene Diagnosis (unmet human need)	Etiology (due to...)	Signs and Symptoms (evidenced by...)	Patient Goals (expected outcomes)
Protection from Health Risks			
Freedom from Fear and Stress			
Freedom from Pain			
Wholesome Facial Image			
Skin and Mucous Membrane Integrity of the Head and Neck			
Biologically Sound and Functional Dentition			
Conceptualization and Problem Solving			
Responsibility for Oral Health			

3 Evidence-Based Decision Making

COMPETENCIES

1. Define evidence-based decision making (EBDM), list the two fundamental principles of EBDM, and discuss evidence sources and levels of evidence.
2. Ask a good PICO question; identify the specific problem, intervention, comparison, and clinical outcome; and conduct a PubMed clinical query to determine if the PICO question efficiently generates relevant, high-quality sources to address the PICO question.
3. Apply the EBDM process and skills to access different sources of evidence, critically appraise and apply it when appropriate, and communicate findings as it relates to providing evidence-based patient care.

SHORT ANSWER QUESTIONS

1. List three examples of secondary research.

_____

_____

_____

_____

_____

_____

2. List two examples observational research.

_____

_____

_____

_____

3. In the PICO Process, PICO stands for:

_____

_____

_____

_____

_____

_____

_____

_____

4. What are the five A's needed to apply the Evidence-Based Decision Making Process?

_____

_____

_____

_____

_____

_____

_____

_____

5. What is the first question that guides the critical analysis process?

_____

_____

_____

_____

_____

FILL IN THE BLANK STATEMENTS

Select the best term from the chapter and complete the following statements.

1. _____ is the use of available evidence together with the clinician's expertise and the patient's preferences in making health care decisions.

2. The model that defines a clinical question in terms of patient problem and aids the researcher in finding clinically relevant evidence in the literature is _____.

3. _____ is a feature of PubMed that provides specialized searches using evidence-based filters to retrieve articles.

4. _____ is a free full-text archive of biomedical and life sciences journal literature.

5. _____ provides systematic reviews of the strongest evidence available concerning health care interventions.

6. _____ includes original studies that can be divided into two categories: experimental studies and observational, studies.

7. A study that strictly adheres to a scientific research design, includes a hypothesis, a variable that can be manipulated by the researcher, and variables that can be measured, calculated, and compared is called _____
_____.

8. A study in which the participants are divided by chance into separate groups that compare different treatments or other interventions is known as a _____.

9. Studies in which the researcher does not give a treatment, intervention, or provide an exposure whereby data are gathered without intervening to control variables is considered a _____
_____.

10. _____ is a research method that involves using information that others have gathered through primary research.

11. _____ summarizes the results of available health care studies and provides a high level of evidence on the effectiveness of health care interventions.

12. _____ is a quantitative epidemiological study design used to systematically assess previous research studies to derive conclusions about that body of research.

13. _____ do not have a research design but incorporates the best available scientific evidence to support a clinical practice.

14. _____ is a measure of whether your research findings are meaningful.

15. _____ distinguishes the importance and meaning of the results reported in a study.

MULTIPLE CHOICE QUESTIONS

Complete each question by circling the best answer.

1. EBDM include all of the following components EXCEPT:
   a. Professional experience
   b. Patient's opinion
   c. ADA reviews
   d. Best available research

2. All of the following will assist in successful PubMed searches EXCEPT:
   a. Start with the PubMed Clinical Queries feature
   b. Maximize search terms to cover all related inquiries
   c. Complete courses on Dentalcare.com
   d. Complete PubMed tutorial

3. Evaluating current research aids in eliminating ineffective past research. Evaluating current research gauges validity of findings as it relates to patient care.
   a. Both statements are true.
   b. Both statements are false.
   c. The first statement is true and the second statement is false.
   d. The first statement is false and the second statement is true.

4. Which item of the PICO process includes the gold standard?
   a. Problem
   b. Intervention
   c. Comparison
   d. Outcome

5. Which of the following is the highest level of evidence?
   a. Randomized control trials
   b. Systematic reviews
   c. Surveys
   d. Clinical practice guidelines

6. Critical summaries are short reviews of the original research. Critical summaries only include an expert commentary on the strengths and weakness of the study.
   a. Both statements are true.
   b. Both statements are false.
   c. The first statement is true and the second statement is false.
   d. The first statement is false and the second statement is true.

7. Which of the following key questions should be asked once the results of a study are valid?
   a. What are the results?
   b. What is the PICO question?
   c. Should the study be repeated?
   d. What is the statistical significance of the study?

8. Statistical significance demonstrates the probability that the results did not occur by chance. Statistical significance has no bearing in clinical implications of the results.
   a. Both statements are true.
   b. Both statements are false.
   c. The first statement is true and the second statement is false.
   d. The first statement is false and the second statement is true.

9. The randomized controlled trial provides the strongest evidence for demonstrating that the treatment has caused the effect, rather than the effect occurring by chance. The randomized controlled trial is considered a primary evidence resource.
   a. Both statements are true.
   b. Both statements are false.
   c. The first statement is true and the second statement is false.
   d. The first statement is false and the second statement is true.

10. Which of the following is the highest level of primary evidence?
    a. National survey
    b. Randomized control trial
    c. Meta-analysis
    d. Cohort studies

Ms. Penelope has been your patient for several years. She has always been a conscious patient always following your professional advice. She is interested in the benefits of oil pulling to reduce gingival inflammation. She has tried to research this topic herself, but she states she gets lost and does not understand the research process.

How do you begin researching oil pulling? Use the PICO model.
What types of research will give you the best information for your patient?

4 Community Health

COMPETENCIES

1. Describe the health care continuum of dental hygiene care and discuss related critical thinking scenarios.
2. Define "health" and discuss health care promotion. Understand that dental hygiene practice, no matter the setting, impacts the client at the individual/family, group, community, and advocacy/policy level.
3. Discuss the concept of the health care continuum and that dental hygienist practice along a continuum of care promoting health and well-being in terms of disease treatment, disease prevention (primary, secondary, and tertiary), and health promotion.
4. Take action and apply health promotion strategies to facilitate client and/or community oral health.

SHORT ANSWER QUESTIONS

1. List several contributors to social determinants of health.

_____

_____

_____

_____

_____

_____

_____

_____

_____

_____

_____

2. Define Health Education.

_____

_____

_____

_____

3. What is the most important aspect of a dental hygienist creating a program for a community?

_____

_____

_____

_____

4. Give an example of a primary prevention dental hygiene intervention.

_____

_____

_____

_____

5. Give an example of a secondary prevention dental hygiene intervention.

_____

_____

_____

_____

6. Give an example of a tertiary prevention dental hygiene intervention.

_____

_____

_____

_____

7. Briefly explain social determinants of health.

_____

_____

_____

_____

FILL IN THE BLANK STATEMENTS

Select the best term from the chapter and complete the following statements.

1. Simplistically, _____ is the absence of disease or infirmity.

2. _____ is the process of enabling people to increase control over and improve their current and future health.

3. Mothers Against Drunk Drivers campaign is an example of _____.

4. _____ is enhancing patients' ability to manage the ever-changing environment.

5. Providing sealants to caries-free children in a Head Start program is an example of _____.

6. Providing sealants to children with insipient caries in a Head Start program is an example of _____.

7. _____ approach focuses on specific needs of a community.

8. Writing an article about early caries prevention in a parenting magazine is an example of _____ influence.

14

Chapter **4** Community Health

Copyright © 2025 by Elsevier Inc. All rights are reserved, including those for text and data mining, AI training, and similar technologies.

9. The social determinants of health require a/an _____ approach that sees the individual existing within a community and _____ contributes to individual health.

10. _____ is learning experiences designed to help individuals and communities improve their health by increasing their knowledge or influencing their attitudes.

MULTIPLE CHOICE QUESTIONS

Complete each question by circling the best answer.

1. All of the following are considered continuum of care promoting health and well-being EXCEPT:
   a. Disease treatment
   b. Health promotion
   c. Health prevention
   d. Disease prevention

2. Disease treatment is a minor aspect of the health continuum of care. The absence of disease is the total definition of health.
   a. Both statements are true.
   b. Both statements are false.
   c. The first statement is true, the second statement is false.
   d. The first statement is false, the second statement is true.

3. All of the following are disease prevention strategies EXCEPT:
   a. Initial
   b. Primary
   c. Secondary
   d. Tertiary

4. Implementing oral cancer screening programs in long term care facilities is an example of what type of prevention?
   a. Initial
   b. Primary
   c. Secondary
   d. Tertiary

5. Advocating with policy makers to fluoridate municipal water is an example of what type of prevention?
   a. Initial
   b. Primary
   c. Secondary
   d. Tertiary

6. The goal of health promotion is to lessen inequities by addressing the determinants of health. The goal of health promotion is to work so that people are more likely to be healthy than to develop disease.
   a. Both statements are true.
   b. Both statements are false.
   c. The first statement is true, the second statement is false.
   d. The first statement is false, the second statement is true.

7. Which if the following is not an example of Interprofessional Collaboration?
   a. Discussing premedication requirements with a physician
   b. Providing athletic guards to a local team of soccer players
   c. Providing education on denture care with nurse's aides
   d. Referring a patient to an endocrinologist for diabetes status changes

8. Educating policy makers on the need for fluoridated community water is an example of:
   a. Change talk
   b. Policy evaluation
   c. Community advocacy
   d. Accountability

9. Sending an email to multiple community members concerning a new program on smoking cessation is an example of:
   a. Health policy
   b. Educational intervention
   c. Mass media
   d. Community involvement

10. Treating periodontal disease is an example of what type of prevention?
    a. Initial
    b. Primary
    c. Secondary
    d. Tertiary

11. Health promotion strategy focuses on:
    a. Community centered initiative
    b. Policy change
    c. Educational involvement
    d. Change talk

12. Dental hygiene association members organized a free sealant day for the local Boys and Girls club. Which health promotion strategy is being used?
    a. Education
    b. Social marketing
    c. Policy change
    d. Community Organization

CASE STUDY

Assess

Diagnose

Plan

Implement

Evaluate

Document

5 | Sustainable Health Behavior Change

COMPETENCIES

1. Discuss extrinsic and intrinsic motivation.
2. Examine motivational interviewing as a client-centered approach to addressing behavior change.
3. List and describe the four core motivational interviewing communication skills.
4. Discuss various communication styles between a client and a health care provider, including guiding, following, and directing.
5. Describe professional dental hygiene relationships, including the PACE principles.
6. Describe factors that inhibit behavior change.
7. Discuss communication with clients throughout the life span.

SHORT ANSWER QUESTIONS

1. What are the three key concepts of extrinsic motivation?

_____

_____

_____

_____

2. List several levels of reflection.

_____

_____

_____

_____

_____

_____

_____

_____

3. Give examples of which physical surroundings may influence with clinician/patient communication.

_____

_____

_____

_____

_____

_____

_____

_____

4. Give examples of which internal psychophysiological factors may influence with clinician/patient communication.

_____

_____

_____

_____

_____

_____

_____

_____

_____

_____

_____

5. What factors inhibit communication?

_____

_____

_____

_____

_____

_____

_____

_____

_____

_____

_____

6. What characteristics do open-ended questions use?

_____

_____

_____

_____

_____

_____

_____

_____

7. If a patient refuses to follow the dental hygienist's oral health recommendation, what ways can the dental hygienist support the patient's decision?

_____

_____

_____

_____

_____

_____

_____

_____

_____

_____

_____

_____

_____

_____

_____

8. List and briefly discuss the mnemonic acronym *PACE*.

_____

_____

_____

_____

FILL IN THE BLANK STATEMENTS

Select the best term from the chapter and complete the following statements.

1. _____ is the ability of the clinician to accept clients as the people they are without allowing any judgment of clients' attitudes or feelings to interfere with communication.

2. _____ are statements made by patients that indicate that they are moving toward making a positive change directed at a problematic behavior.

3. _____ allow for only a limited or narrow answer to an inquiry.

4. _____ is action initiated from an environmental source.

5. A _____ is a technique used by the clinician to listen actively and empathetically as well as to understand patient's problems or concerns.

6. _____ is a behavior that comes from within an individual whereby no external rewards are required and the behavior itself is the reward.

7. _____ is a counseling method that helps patients change an undesired behavior to find the internal motivation they need to change that behavior.

MULTIPLE CHOICE QUESTIONS

Complete each question by circling the best answer.

1. "Tell me about other health issues you are concerned about" is an example of what type of open-ended questioning a dental hygienist might pose?
   a. Clarifying
   b. Testing
   c. Directive
   d. Developmental

2. All of the following cultural context factors may influence with clinician/patient communication EXCEPT:
   a. Emotional status
   b. Language
   c. Education
   d. Customs

3. All of the following are components of Havinghurst's Adult Developmental middle age stage EXCEPT:
   a. Meeting social and civic obligations
   b. Developing durable leisure-time activities
   c. Relating to one's marriage partner as a person
   d. Accepting and adjusting to physical change

4. "From what you've said, you don't think you can return for 4-month recare visits due to finances, is that correct?" This is an example of what type of open-ended questioning a dental hygienist might pose?
   a. Clarifying
   b. Testing
   c. Directive
   d. Developmental

5. All of the following are situational context factors may influence with clinician/patient communication EXCEPT:
   a. Goal attainment
   b. Self-esteem
   c. Problem solving
   d. Expression of feelings

6. Which of the following statements is true concerning open-ended questioning?
   a. Leads the patient in discussing chief complaints
   b. Informs the patient that HIPAA is observed to protect their opinions
   c. Encourages short answers to be mindful of treatment time
   d. Begins with *what, how or why*?

7. Which term best represents the clinician repeating or restating a patient's concern?
   a. Paraphrasing
   b. Change talk
   c. Extrinsic motivation
   d. Acceptance

CASE STUDY: MR. ROSE

Mr. Rose is 35 years old and has been a patient in your practice for over 10 years. He is diligent with his homecare and is consistent with 6-month appointments. Mr. Rose smokes 1½ packs of cigarettes a day and has smoked for 20 years. Recent changes in his health history reveal hypertension. He also has family history of coronary heart disease. He admitted to drinking 2–3 beers a night. His periodontal condition has slightly declined over the past year. You discussed smoking cessation with him several years ago, and he became annoyed and asked that you not bring up the subject again. You feel that due to changes in his medical history, oral health, and overall health, it is in his best interest to revisit the subject again. What specific strategies do you use to assist him in his behavior change?

6 | Inclusive Practices in Healthcare

COMPETENCIES

1. Discuss the relationship between culture and health, and work toward developing cultural sensitivity through self-awareness and exploration of cultural self-identify and identity of others.
2. Understand the relationship between cultural competence, cultural humility, and patient-centered care.
3. Describe health care literacy and value the importance of cultural values, health beliefs, and cultural sensitivity.
4. Value the importance of verbal, nonverbal, and written communication utilizing Motivational Interviewing techniques and LEARN frameworks to communicate with patients in inclusive encounters.
5. Discuss the importance of cultural sensitivity when making shared decisions in the health care environment.
6. Discuss the process of care in patient-centered environments.

SHORT ANSWER QUESTIONS

1. What is the LEARN model?

_____

_____

_____

_____

_____

_____

_____

_____

_____

_____

2. What is the ETHNIC Model?

_____

_____

_____

_____

_____

_____

_____

_____

_____

_____

_____

_____

3. List approaches the dental hygienist should do when providing patient education in a cross-cultural environment.

_____

_____

_____

_____

_____

_____

4. List characteristics of communication that maximizes effective cross-cultural communication.

_____

_____

_____

_____

_____

_____

_____

_____

5. What are the five constructs of the Process of Cultural Competence in the Delivery of Healthcare Services Model?

_____

_____

_____

_____

_____

_____

_____

_____

_____

6. What are the goals and intentions of the National Standards for Culturally and Linguistically Appropriate Services (CLAS) in Health and Health Care?

_____

_____

_____

_____

_____

_____

_____

FILL IN THE BLANK STATEMENTS

Select the best term from the chapter and complete the following statements.

1. _____ is the degree to which a patient has the capacity to obtain, process, and understand health information and services needed to make appropriate health decisions in a particular language.

2. _____ is the awareness and sensitivity that cultural differences and similarities exist can affect values, learning, and behavior.

3. _____ is the ability to conduct a cultural and physical assessment to collect relevant cultural data regarding the patients' chief compliant.

4. _____ is the often erroneous assumption that a person possesses certain characteristics or traits simply because he or she is a member of a particular group.

5. _____ is the belief that one's culture is superior to another's culture.

6. _____ is the process of self-examination and self-assessment of one's own culture and its potential influence on one's ways of thinking and behaving.

7. _____ is the information one knows about cultures including the cultural history, values, beliefs, characteristics, and behaviors of another ethnic or cultural group.

8. _____ is knowledge and understanding of another person's culture allowing one to better adapt interventions and approaches to health care to the specific culture of the patient, family, and social group.

9. _____ is a group of people who have developed interests or goals different from the primary culture.

10. _____ is a set of guidelines that one can inherit as a member of a group or society and may influence the way the members of that society or group view the world.

MULTIPLE CHOICE QUESTIONS

Complete each question by circling the best answer.

1. Your new patient, Celeste Moon, arrives for dental hygiene treatment. She has many visible tattoos and piercings and is carrying a bag that says, "Save the Earth." Before she even sits in your chair, you suspect she will have poor hygiene, periodontal disease, and rampant decay. You also suspect she will refuse radiographs and think fluoride is poison. This preconceived attitude is an example of:
   a. Cultural sensitivity
   b. Stereotyping
   c. Ethnocentrism
   d. Cultural incompetence

2. Cultural competency is attaining knowledge and understanding of another person's culture. Cultural competency adapts interventions and approaches to health care to the specific culture of the dental hygienist.
   a. Both statements are true.
   b. Both statements are false.
   c. The first statement is true and the second statement is false.
   d. The first statement is false and the second statement is true.

3. A group of people who develop interests that are different from their primary group is:
   a. Cultural sensitivity
   b. Cultural skill
   c. Culture shock
   d. Subculture

4. Poverty is often the reason a patient does not seek dental care. Unemployment often a barrier to patients meeting their basic human need for overall health and oral health.
   a. Both statements are true.
   b. Both statements are false.
   c. The first statement is true and the second statement is false.
   d. The first statement is false and the second statement is true.

5. All of the following forms of nonverbal communication can be a source of miscommunication in cross-cultural encounters EXCEPT:
   a. Hand gestures
   b. Facial expressions
   c. Physical contact
   d. Eye contact

6. All of the following are Social Determinants of Health EXCEPT:
   a. Economic stability
   b. Health and Healthcare
   c. Social and Community Context
   d. Access to care

7. In an individualistic environment, a single person is central decision maker with autonomy and self-determination as an essential element to make medical and dental care decisions. In a collectivist environment, the group is viewed as the fundamental unit of society and the group is seen as the decision maker for medical and dental care decisions.
   a. Both statements are true.
   b. Both statements are false.
   c. The first statement is true and the second statement is false.
   d. The first statement is false and the second statement is true.

8. What is the most important component when using the LEARN model for communicating in cross-cultural environments?
   a. Passive learning
   b. Active learning
   c. Passive listening
   d. Active listening

9. Providing culturally sensitive oral health care begins with which person?
   a. Patient's primary care physician
   b. Receptionist who makes the first patient contact
   c. Patient's family member or friend
   d. Clinician providing treatment

10. All of the following consequences of ineffective communication caused by cultural differences between the clinician and the patient EXCEPT:
    a. Clinician dissatisfaction
    b. Decreased trust
    c. Adherence to recommendations
    d. Adverse health outcomes

11. Which recent but ongoing paradigm combines cultural competence with cultural humility?
    a. Classism
    b. Cultural encounter
    c. Cultural competemility
    d. Cultural ability

25

Your new patient presents to the office for routine care. She is Navajo and speaks no English. She has never had her teeth professionally cleaned. She arrives with an interpreter who assists you in understanding the culture of the Navajo. The interpreter gives you some basic information concerning Navajo culture and health care:

They believe in the concept of "Hozho," which embraces goodness, harmony, positive attitude, and universal beauty. Any kind of illness is thought to be a disruption of Hozho, and discussion of illness conflicts with this philosophy. Direct eye contact is frowned upon. Instead of firm handshaking during greetings, touching of hands is used instead. Navajo also believe that traditional healers already know the patient's health conditions and some interview questions may seem unnecessary.

Navajo health culture also believes diseases are said to be caused by forbidden behavior or by sick/infected animals. Radiographs are believed to be linked to the patient's soul. It may be beneficial to ask the patient if she would like additional assistance from a traditional Navajo healer, as it may help improve cooperation with the recommendations. Use third-party references when discussing negative information, such as "some people have gum disease." Frame all health discussions in a positive way.

How do you proceed with your initial assessment? What are your recommendations? Develop a dental hygiene care plan for Mrs. N.

Age	60	SCENARIO
Gender	female	**EOE/IOE:** Fissured tongue Moderate biofilm generalized Moderate calculus generalized
Height	5'2"	
Weight	120 lb	
B/P	120/70 mm Hg	**Periodontal Findings:** 3-4 mm pockets generalized Moderate inflammation generalized
Chief Complaint	Pain in maxillary right quadrant. Recommended to have her oral health evaluated from Nurse practitioner who recently visited to her village	**Radiographic Findings:** Caries present on tooth #2,3,14,19,30
Medical History	Severe arthritis in hands and feet	
Current Medications	Herbal remedies from her Navajo healer	
Social History		

Using the data from this patient, develop a Human Needs Conceptual model for treatment.

Dental Hygiene Diagnosis (unmet human need)	Etiology (due to...)	Signs and Symptoms (evidenced by...)	Patient Goals (expected outcomes)
Protection from Health Risks			
Freedom from Fear and Stress			
Freedom from Pain			
Wholesome Facial Image			
Skin and Mucous Membrane Integrity of the Head and Neck			
Biologically Sound and Functional Dentition			
Conceptualization and Problem Solving			
Responsibility for Oral Health			

7 Legal and Ethical Decision Making

COMPETENCIES

1. Demonstrate an understanding of the dental hygiene codes of ethics and key ethical principles given ethical scenarios.
2. Apply the ethical decision-making framework to resolve ethical dilemmas encountered in practice.
3. Explain the ethical challenges of the dental hygienist–patient relationship, the dental hygienist–dental hygienist relationship, and the employer-employee relationship. Also, discuss the usage of a dental ethics committee.
4. Discuss and describe the basic legal concepts, contract and tort principles, and risk management strategies that affect oral health professionals.
5. Explain legal concepts in the dental hygienist–patient relationship, the dental hygienist-dentist relationship, and employer-employee relationship.
6. Suggest risk management strategies to reduce legal risks and liabilities of dental hygienists engaged in various roles.
7. Describe ethical dilemmas, legal issues, and roles of the dental hygienist as a dependent and independent clinical practitioner, independent contractor, administrator or manager, educator, consumer advocate, and public health professional.

SHORT ANSWER QUESTIONS

1. Name the three colleague relationships that a code of ethics recognizes.

_____

_____

_____

_____

_____

2. List and briefly describe the fundamental ethical principles.

_____

_____

_____

_____

_____

_____

3. List the Ethical Decision-Making Framework.

_____

_____

_____

_____

_____

_____

4. Identify common dental malpractice litigations.

_____

_____

_____

_____

_____

_____

_____

5. Name the two categories of the law.

_____

_____

_____

6. Explain the difference between an implied contract and an express contract.

_____

_____

_____

_____

7. Briefly describe the two types of torts.

_____

_____

_____

_____

_____

_____

8. Failure to meet the standard of care in dental hygiene may include what?

_____

_____

_____

_____

_____

_____

9. List the information a patient should be told to attain informed consent.

_____

_____

_____

_____

_____

_____

_____

_____

_____

_____

10. List information that an informed refusal form should include.

_____

_____

_____

_____

_____

_____

_____

11. Briefly explain confidentiality.

_____

_____

_____

_____

_____

12. Briefly describe the two types of defamation.

_____

_____

_____

13. List items on an employment application that are unlawful.

_____

_____

_____

_____

_____

_____

_____

_____

_____

_____

_____

_____

_____

_____

FILL IN THE BLANK STATEMENTS

Select the best term from the chapter and complete the following statements.

1. A situation whereby two ethical principles are in conflict is a(n) _____.

2. In a lawsuit, the _____ is the person who files the suit.

3. In a lawsuit, the _____ is the person denying the action charged.

4. A _____ may outline specific conditions or obligations that must be satisfied by the patient and the provider.

5. Practitioner-patient relationship terminated without giving the patient adequate notice or time to locate another practitioner is _____.

6. A __ is an interference with another's right to enjoy person, privacy, or property.

7. _____ is the degree of care a reasonably prudent professional would exercise under the same or similar circumstances.

8. _____ is a process whereby a patient voluntarily agrees to proposed treatment after a discussion of advantages, disadvantages, risks, and alternatives.

9. _____ is a person's right to refuse any or all of a proposed treatment after the recommended treatment, alternate treatment options, and the possible consequences of declining treatment have been explained in a language the patient understands.

10. A _____ is the length of time an aggrieved person has to enter lawsuits against another for an alleged injury.

11. A _____ is recommended to identify potential risks in the delivery of oral care.

MULTIPLE CHOICE QUESTIONS

Complete each question by circling the best answer.

1. Financial reimbursements received from patients with Medicaid are much less than financial reimbursements received from patients with private insurance. Office policy for Molar Dental Office is to schedule 30 minutes for routine dental hygiene care for a patient with Medicaid and 60 minutes for routine care for a patient with private insurance. What ethical principle does this exemplify?
   a. Beneficence
   b. Maleficence
   c. Justice
   d. Fidelity

2. When entering a contractual agreement with a health care provider, the patient's only responsibility is to pay the agreed-upon fees for services. The health care provider may dismiss a patient from the practice for failing to disclose vital health information.
   a. Both statements are true.
   b. Both statements are false.
   c. The first statement is true, the second statement is false.
   d. The first statement is false, the second statement is true.

3. Your patient is a very cooperative 9-year-old boy. His lower right lateral incisor is very loose and will naturally exfoliate within a week. He asks you to please remove his tooth so the Tooth Fairy can visit him that night. His mother gives you permission, and you place topical anesthesia on the surrounding tissue, grasp the tooth with a gauze, and twist the tooth out. What ethical principle does this exemplify, if any?
   a. Beneficence
   b. Maleficence
   c. Nonmaleficence
   d. There is no ethical dilemma. No instruments were used and the parent gave consent.

4. An implied contract has no written documentation of agreement; however, a contractual relationship exists. An express contract expresses terms in either a verbal or a written agreement.
   a. Both statements are true.
   b. Both statements are false.
   c. The first statement is true, the second statement is false.
   d. The first statement is false, the second statement is true.

5. Your 75-year-old patient requires quadrant scaling/periodontal therapy. She understands and would like to proceed with treatment; however, her adult daughter insists that the treatment is not necessary and losing teeth at her mother's age is normal. What ethical principal does this violate for your patient?
   a. Beneficence
   b. Maleficence
   c. Justice
   d. Autonomy

6. Criminal law addresses behavior that is an offense against the public, society, or the state while civil law addresses behavior that constitutes an injury to an individual.
   a. Both parts of the statement are true.
   b. Both parts of the statement are false.
   c. The first part is true, the second is false.
   d. The first part is false, the second is true.

7. Your local dental hygiene association has initiated a sealant day for at-risk children. What ethical principle does this represent?
   a. Beneficence
   b. Maleficence
   c. Veracity
   d. Autonomy

8. For a civil act, the level of proof required is that beyond a reasonable doubt. For a criminal act, the level of proof required is a preponderance of evidence.
   a. Both statements are true.
   b. Both statements are false.
   c. The first statement is true, the second statement is false.
   d. The first statement is false, the second statement is true.

9. Your patient is interested in quitting smoking. Your office provides free bleaching when he maintains 3 months being smoke free. What ethical principle does this represent?
   a. Fidelity
   b. Maleficence
   c. Veracity
   d. Autonomy

10. Your last patient of the day, a 25-year-old female, is new to the practice. She reports not having any dental or dental hygiene treatment in over 3 years. Periodontal findings indicate 2-3 mm pocket depths with slight inflammation, Type I periodontal classification. You inform your patient that she needs four quadrants periodontal scaling and you will complete two quadrants that day. Since you have a daily production quota to meet, this treatment will satisfy the quota. What ethical principle does this represent?
    a. Fidelity
    b. Maleficence
    c. Veracity
    d. Autonomy

11. Libel is written defamation. Slander is verbal defamation.
    a. Both statements are true.
    b. Both statements are false.
    c. The first statement is true, the second statement is false.
    d. The first statement is false, the second statement is true.

12. The Age Discrimination in Employment Act of 1967 (ADEA) is a local law that affects employers with 10 or more employees. The act prohibits discrimination on the basis of age between 40 and 70 years.
    a. Both statements are true.
    b. Both statements are false.
    c. The first statement is true, the second statement is false.
    d. The first statement is false, the second statement is true.

13. The Americans with Disabilities Act (ADA) prohibits employment discrimination against qualified individuals with disabilities. An individual qualifies for protection under this act if he or she has a physical or mental impairment that substantially limits one or more major life activities.
    a. Both statements are true.
    b. Both statements are false.
    c. The first statement is true, the second statement is false.
    d. The first statement is false, the second statement is true.

14. The Equal Pay Act of 1963 protects men and women who perform substantially equal work in the same establishment from gender-based wage discrimination. The law would allow an employer to reduce the wages of either a man or a woman to equalize inequities in pay.
    a. Both statements are true.
    b. Both statements arc false.
    c. The first statement is true, the second statement is false.
    d. The first statement is false, the second statement is true.

15. Quid pro quo involves a superior-subordinate relationship in which the offender has control over the working conditions of the victim. Hostile environment includes unwelcome, demeaning verbal or physical conduct of a sexual nature that creates a hostile, intimidating, or offensive work environment.
    a. Both statements are true.
    b. Both statements are false.
    c. The first statement is true, the second statement is false.
    d. The first statement is false, the second statement is true

CASE STUDY

1. You are logged in to a social media site and you come across an advertisement for bleaching at a very low cost. You notice the person offering this service is a dental hygienist working out of a nail salon. Using the following steps, how would you approach this dilemma?

   a. Define the conflict or dilemma

   _____

   _____

   _____

   _____

   _____

   b. Identify the ethical issue

   _____

   _____

   _____

   c. Gather relevant information

   _____

   _____

   _____

   d. Identify the ethical alternatives

   _____

   _____

   _____

   e. Establish an ethical position and prioritize alternatives

   _____

   _____

   _____

   f. Select, justify, and defend the chosen alternative

   _____

   _____

   _____

   g. Act on the ethical choice

   _____

   _____

   _____

8 Professional e-Portfolios

COMPETENCIES

1. Differentiate between the various types and formats of portfolios and their uses.
2. Describe the process for creating a student portfolio and identify artifacts or projects that would demonstrate competency.
3. Examine the role of reflection within the portfolio.
4. Discuss the role that ethics plays in portfolio authorship.
5. Describe how the student portfolio can be transitioned for use throughout the career of the dental hygienist.

SHORT ANSWER QUESTIONS

1. Which state was the first to accept a hybrid portfolio for initial licensure in dentistry?

_____

_____

_____

_____

2. What activity may enhance reflective writing in the student portfolio?

_____

_____

_____

_____

3. Which ethical principle applies to creating a professional portfolio?

_____

_____

4. What components should be included in the biographical data section when compiling a professional portfolio?

_____

_____

_____

5. What artifacts should be included in an e-portfolio?

_____

_____

_____

_____

6. Write a reflection statement on a clinical experience that challenged you.

_____

_____

_____

_____

FILL IN THE BLANK STATEMENTS

Select the best term from the chapter and complete the following statements.

1. A physical collection of carefully selected items that demonstrate professional accomplishments and growth is a

_____.

2. _____ is a collection of academic works that have been organized to demonstrate progressive learning, academic achievement, and evidence of meeting institutional standards or course requirements.

3. The _____ is a collection of academic works that demonstrates progressive learning and evidence of meeting or exceeding clinical competence.

4. _____ is an expansion of a resume and is used by professionals to illustrate accomplishments, skills, and relevant experiences.

5. The _____ is usually organized in binders or folders whereas the _____ is often web-based and stored virtually.

6. A _____ is a written expression that reviews an event and allows the writer a greater understanding of self and to critically evaluate performance to enhance future learning.

MULTIPLE CHOICE QUESTIONS

Complete each question by circling the best answer.

1. Professional portfolios are used for employment for all of the following EXCEPT:
   a. Visual record of the candidate's abilities and accomplishments
   b. Marketing tool to potential employers
   c. Visual prompt in the interview process
   d. Initial government application

2. Current portfolio formats include all of the following EXCEPT:
   a. Paper
   b. Video
   c. Electronic

3. What key component in a portfolio adds richness and depth?
   a. Clinical effectiveness
   b. Research papers
   c. Community projects
   d. Reflection

4. A résumé is a brief document summarizing education, employment history, and experiences relevant to a specific employment position. A curriculum vitae is an ongoing overview of professional activities documenting employment, education, teaching, publications, honors, and volunteer activities.
   a. Both statements are true.
   b. Both statements are false.
   c. The first statement is true, the second statement is false.
   d. The first statement is false, the second statement is true.

5. Who is responsible for updating and maintaining state licensure requirements for licensees?
   a. State Board of Dentistry
   b. Licensed professional
   c. Dental hygiene school administrator
   d. CODA

6. Which document is a brief account of an individual's education, employment history, experiences related to specific employment positions, and a cover letter?
   a. CV
   b. Reflection statement
   c. Resume
   d. Portfolio

7. Which document is an ongoing record of education, employment, teaching positions, publications, volunteer activities, and honors?
   a. CV
   b. Resume
   c. Portfolio
   d. Artifacts

Dental Hygiene Patient Care Settings

COMPETENCIES

1. Discuss the equipment and areas included in a patient treatment area in a dental/dental hygiene office or clinic.
2. Compare and contrast the dental hygiene care environment in a dental office, college or university, and correctional facility to include the components of the dental hygiene treatment area.
3. Apply knowledge of the dental hygiene care environment unique to a correctional facility and an institutionalized setting and delivery of patient care services in that setting.
4. Explain the adjustments that a dental hygiene care provider must consider when delivering services in a school-based oral health prevention program, mobile dental facility, or outreach settings using teledentistry. Also, describe the influence of patient setting on the dental hygiene care environment.

SHORT ANSWER QUESTIONS

1. Describe the dental delivery system.

_____

_____

_____

_____

2. List various settings for dental hygiene clinical practice.

_____

_____

_____

_____

_____

_____

3. What is the difference between a saddle stool, an operator stool, and a dental assistant stool?

_____

_____

_____

_____

_____

4. Which government agency has standards set for water used in routine dental treatment?

_____

_____

_____

_____

5. Which government agency sets the standards for dental devices connected to a water system?

_____

_____

FILL IN THE BLANK STATEMENTS

Select the best term from the chapter and complete the following statements.

1. The sterilization area is also known as _____.

2. The area for construction of study models, adjustment of dental appliances, fabrication of mouth guards, and custom fluoride or whitening trays is the _____.

3. _____ is the physical setting that contains equipment and instruments where the dental hygienist delivers professional oral care.

4. In accordance with _____, the clerical area should remain private to allow for exchange of confidential information.

5. _____ and _____ lines assist with patient rinsing and maintain visibility and a dry field during care.

6. Dental radiographs may be either _____ or _____ format.

MULTIPLE CHOICE QUESTIONS

Complete each question by circling the best answer.

1. All of the following are methods for contaminated instrument sterilization EXCEPT:
   a. Ultrasonic instrument cleaning device
   b. Dry heat sterilizer
   c. Steam pressure sterilizer
   d. Chemical device

2. Which government agency sets the standards for water quality in the dental hygiene care environment?
   a. CDC
   b. EPA
   c. OSHA
   d. FDA

3. The dental setting that accommodates a simulation lab is:
   a. Educational setting
   b. Correctional facility
   c. Institutionalized setting
   d. Mobile dental facility

4. The dental setting that has only instruments and equipment necessary to provide treatment is:
   a. Institutionalized setting
   b. School-based oral health programs
   c. Mobile dental facility
   d. Correctional facility

5. Which setting would the dental hygienist provide services to a patient who has medically complex needs?
   a. Educational setting
   b. Correctional facility
   c. Institutionalized setting
   d. Mobile dental facility

6. School-based oral health programs provide certain preventive services to at-risk populations. The most common services provided are exams, radiographs, and simple restorations.
   a. Both statements are true.
   b. Both statements are false.
   c. The first statement is true, the second statement is false.
   d. The first statement is false, the second statement is true.

7. A mobile dental facility will include:
   a. Clerical area
   b. Dark room
   c. Dental lab
   d. Treatment area

8. Reaching out to underserved in remote populations to provide oral care using dental professionals and technology is:
   a. Educational setting
   b. Correctional facility
   c. Institutionalized setting
   d. Mobile dental facility

9. Which setting became most popular during the COVID-19 pandemic?
   a. Mobile dental facility
   b. Educational setting
   c. Teledentistry
   d. Academic setting

10. Which dental setting offers services that include sealants, fluoride treatments, and oral health education?
    a. Institutional
    b. School-based
    c. Military-based
    d. Teledentistry

10 Infection Prevention and Control

COMPETENCIES

1. Discuss standard precautions and basic infection-control concepts.
2. Explain the similarities and differences between the infection-control model and model of dental hygiene care.
3. Identify the government agencies that play key roles in regulations of infection control standards.
4. Discuss the standard of care, including assessment of risk of disease transmission in oral health care, and planning of appropriate control measures.
5. Explain the principles of infection control, including:
   - Select appropriate protective attire for dental hygiene patient care.
   - Prepare the dental environment before and after patient care.
6. Discuss strategies to prevent disease transmission, and how health care personnel can take action to stay healthy.

SHORT ANSWER QUESTIONS

1. Which government agency's mission is to apply disease prevention and control, environmental health, and health promotion and health education activities designed to improve the health of the people of the US?

   _____

   _____

   _____

   _____

2. What government agency's mission is to assure safe and healthful working conditions for working men and women by setting and enforcing standards and by providing training, outreach, education, and assistance?

   _____

   _____

   _____

   _____

3. What are the effective goals in the infection control model?

   _____

   _____

   _____

   _____

   _____

4. List how organisms can be transmitted in the dental setting and give examples of each.

_____

_____

_____

_____

_____

_____

_____

_____

_____

_____

5. Briefly describe the chain of infection.

_____

_____

_____

_____

_____

_____

6. List the types of recommended hand hygiene.

_____

_____

_____

_____

_____

7. List the two most common spores that are used in biological indicators.

_____

_____

_____

_____

_____

8. List examples of infection control measures that reduce the spread of contamination.

_____

_____

_____

_____

_____

_____

_____

_____

_____

9. What is a written program that identifies the specific steps to follow after an exposure incident and includes training and education regarding the types of exposure that put DHCP at risk and procedures for prompt reporting and evaluation?

_____

_____

10. List the two objectives of infection prevention and control in the dental setting.

_____

_____

_____

FILL IN THE BLANK STATEMENTS

Select the best term from the chapter and complete the following statements.

1. The mission of _____ is to promote health and quality of life by preventing and controlling disease, injury, and disability.

2. _____ enforces workplace safety regulations, including those for infection control in health care settings.

3. _____ are the infection prevention and control practices whereby health care workers follow the same protocols for all patients regardless of infectious status or health history.

4. _____ is the destruction of all living organisms, including highly resistant bacterial spores.

5. _____ are instruments that penetrate soft tissue or bone.

6. _____ are not intended to penetrate soft tissue or bone but contact oral fluids.

7. _____ are those items that come into contact only with intact skin.

8. _____ uses high heat, whereby temperatures often reach 350°F for a specific amount of time to achieve sterile results.

9. _____ such as floors, walls, and sinks may become contaminated during patient care, but carry less risk of disease transmission than clinical contact surfaces.

10. _____ are surfaces that become contaminated from spray or droplets of oral fluids or by touching with gloved hands during the procedure.

11. An _____ occur when an infectious disease spreads rapidly and affects a greater number of people than generally expected within a given population.

12. A_____ occurs when an epidemic spreads worldwide.

13. The goal of _____ is to prevent health care–associated infections among patients and injuries and illnesses in dental health care personnel.

MULTIPLE CHOICE QUESTIONS

Complete each question by circling the best answer.

1. All of the following government agencies are integral to setting guidelines and regulations for infection control in clinical dental settings EXCEPT:
   a. ADA
   b. CDC
   c. EPA
   d. OSHA

2. The infection control model is designed to:
   a. Protect both the health care provider and the patient
   b. Determine degree of risk a patient has for infection
   c. Protect the health care provider
   d. Protect the patient

3. Chemical indicators signify effectiveness of sterilization. Biological indicators ensure the highest level of sterility.
   a. Both statements are true.
   b. Both statements are false.
   c. The first statement is true, the second statement is false.
   d. The first statement is false, the second statement is true.

4. The CDC develops guidelines and recommendations for practice in the health care setting. The CDC is a regulatory agency that enforces the guidelines and recommendations.
   a. Both statements are true.
   b. Both statements are false.
   c. The first statement is true, the second statement is false.
   d. The first statement is false, the second statement is true.

5. A biological indicator provides information on whether necessary conditions were met to kill a specified number of microorganisms for a given sterilization process. Bacterial spores are the microorganisms primarily used in biological indicators and are considered the most resistant to kill.
   a. Both statements are true.
   b. Both statements are false.
   c. The first statement is true, the second statement is false.
   d. The first statement is false, the second statement is true.

6. Which of the following is the mission of the FDA?
   a. To monitor products for continued safety after they are in use
   b. To obtain accurate, science-based information needed to improve health
   c. To promote health and quality of life by preventing and controlling disease, injury, and disability
   d. To protect human health and the environment

7. Organization for Safety Asepsis and Prevention (OSAP) provides credible resources and tools for Infection Prevention and Control in Dentistry. American National Standards Institute (ANSI) provides standards for protective clothing and eyewear.
   a. Both statements are true.
   b. Both statements are false.
   c. The first statement is true, the second statement is false.
   d. The first statement is false, the second statement is true.

8. CDC recommends all of the following immunizations for health care workers EXCEPT:
   a. Varicella
   b. Hepatitis B
   c. Hepatitis A
   d. Influenza

9. Which of the following is considered a critical instrument?
   a. Instrument tray
   b. Digital x-ray sensors
   c. Mouth mirror
   d. Columbia 13/14 curet

10. When should post-exposure prophylaxis treatment of potential HIV exposure begin?
   a. Under 1 hour post-exposure
   b. 1-2 hours post-exposure
   c. 3-6 hours post-exposure
   d. 7-24 hours post-exposure

11. Which of the following is considered a semicritical instrument?
   a. Shepherd's hook explorer
   b. Impression tray
   c. Light handle
   d. Gracey ½

12. Which method of sterilization monitoring ensures proper sterilization of dental instruments?
    a. Visual
    b. Mechanical
    c. Chemical
    d. Biological

13. Which of the following is the purpose of standard precautions?
    a. Determine a patient's transmission-based risk of infection
    b. Evaluate a patient's health history to determine risk of infection
    c. Infection control practices that follow the same protocols for all patients
    d. Identify possible causes of risk of infection

11 Preventing and Managing Medical Emergencies

COMPETENCIES

1. Prepare the dental team and dental environment to prevent and manage a medical emergency.
2. Discuss the importance of documentation in relation to medical emergencies.
3. Understand the role of anxiety in dental treatment and emergencies.
4. Describe responses to and management of medical emergencies.
5. Recognize necessary legal considerations for medical emergencies.

SHORT ANSWER QUESTIONS

1. List basic medications, equipment, and supplies of a basic dental emergency kit.

_____

_____

_____

_____

_____

_____

_____

_____

_____

_____

_____

_____

_____

_____

2. Briefly describe the ASA Classifications.

_____

_____

_____

_____

_____

_____

3. Describe the symptoms of anaphylaxis.

_____

_____

_____

_____

_____

_____

_____

_____

_____

_____

4. What are the five links in the chain of survival during a life-threatening emergency?

_____

_____

_____

_____

_____

_____

_____

_____

_____

_____

_____

5. Your patient's blood pressure reading is 190/130 mm Hg. What is your plan to avoid a medical emergency?

_____

_____

_____

_____

_____

_____

FILL IN THE BLANK STATEMENTS

Select the best term from the chapter and complete the following statements.

1. _____ is the level of medical care or intervention used for victims of life-threatening illnesses or injuries until they can be given full medical care at a health care facility.

2. An emergency procedure that is performed to manually preserve brain function until further actions are taken to restore spontaneous blood circulation and breathing in a person who is not breathing, not breathing normally (only gasping), and/or has no pulse is _____.

3. The measured percentage of hemoglobin-binding sites in the bloodstream occupied by oxygen is called _____ _____.

4. _____ is a medical device that indirectly monitors the oxygen saturation of a patient's blood and changes in blood volume in the skin.

5. _____ is a temporary loss of consciousness usually related to insufficient blood flow to the brain and most often occurs when blood pressure drops suddenly, and the heart doesn't pump enough oxygen to the brain.

6. A legal term that refers to someone who renders aid in an emergency to an injured person on a voluntary basis is referred to as a _____.

MULTIPLE CHOICE QUESTIONS

Complete each question by circling the best answer.

1. All dental offices should include IV medications used for advanced life support in their emergency kit. All dental offices should include opioid or benzodiazepine reversal drugs in their emergency kit.
   a. Both statements are true.
   b. Both statements are false.
   c. The first statement is true and the second statement is false.
   d. The first statement is false and the second statement is true.

2. Your patient appears cyanotic and is having difficulty breathing. You notice her ankles are swollen, she is perspiring, and her sputum is pink and frothy. This condition is most likely:
   a. Grand mal seizure
   b. Cardiac arrest
   c. Arterial hemorrhage
   d. Pulmonary edema

3. One major cause of vasodepressor syncope in dental settings is:
   a. Allergic reaction to local anesthetic
   b. Diabetes-related crisis
   c. Cardiovascular disease
   d. Fear and anxiety

4. Your patient recently had a myocardial infarction. What ASA classification this patient?
   a. I
   b. II
   c. III
   d. IV

5. All of the following direct observations are present in an anxious patient EXCEPT:
   a. Increased heart rate
   b. Sweating
   c. Pinpoint pupils
   d. Extreme uneasiness

6. All of the following are important in preventing a medical emergency EXCEPT:
   a. All clinicians must be CPR certified
   b. Comprehensive and updated medical history
   c. Vital signs
   d. Medications

7. Your notice your patient has subtle muscle twitching, has a brief blank stare, and appears to be daydreaming for several seconds. This condition is most likely:
   a. Cerebral hypoxia
   b. Hypoglycemia
   c. CVA
   d. Petit mal seizure

8. During treatment, you notice your patient's skin becomes dry and flushed. You retake her vital signs and find she has a weak, rapid pulse. Her breathing is labored, and she has a fruity smell to her breath. What condition has most likely occurred?
   a. Hypoglycemia
   b. Ketoacidosis
   c. Severe anxiety
   d. TIA

9. Your 18-year-old patient is pregnant. She is otherwise very healthy. What is her ASA classification?
   a. I
   b. II
   c. III
   d. IV

10. Your patient accidently inhaled a cotton roll during treatment. He is coughing and trying to dislodge the cotton roll himself. What is you FIRST course of emergency management?
    a. Activate EMS
    b. Encourage the patient to continue coughing to dislodge the object and clear the airway
    c. Sit the patient upright and begin the Heimlich maneuver until the cotton roll is dislodged
    d. Use chest compressions until the cotton roll is dislodged

11. Your anxious patient reports being nauseous. He is perspiring, his pupils are dilated, and he loses consciousness. You patient most likely:
    a. Experienced an aura
    b. Has hypoglycemia
    c. Had a petit mal seizure
    d. Fainted

12. As you are conducting your extra-intraoral exam, your patient's lips, tongue, larynx, and pharynx begin to swell. You conclude that she is allergic to your latex exam gloves. She becomes unresponsive. What is you FIRST course of emergency management?
    a. Activate EMS
    b. Administer O_2 as needed
    c. Administer Epi Pen
    d. Place the patient in a supine position

13. You administered local anesthesia in preparation for SCRP. Your patient's respiration increases, and he states he is lightheaded. He is able to respond to your questions. You perform all of the following EXCEPT:
    a. Activate EMS
    b. Monitor vital signs
    c. Position comfortably
    d. Initiate CPR

14. You begin taking radiographs, and your patient states he is having crushing pain in his chest and mandible. You notice he has shortness of breath and has begun to perspire. His health history was negative for history of cardiovascular abnormalities. What is you FIRST course of emergency management?
    a. Initiate CPR
    b. Monitor vital signs
    c. Administer vasoconstrictor
    d. Activate EMS

15. Your patient begins to cough uncontrollably, wheeze, and efforts to breathe are labored. Your patient has a history of asthma. You perform all of the following EXCEPT:
    a. Have patient administer bronchodilator
    b. Administer CPR
    c. Assess and maintain airway
    d. Stop dental hygiene services

16. During treatment, your patient tells you he has a severe headache, then begins to have difficulty speaking. What condition has most likely occurred?
    a. CVA
    b. Cardiac arrest
    c. Angina pectoris
    d. Adrenal crisis

17. Your anxious patient begins to hyperventilate during treatment. You provide all of the following EXCEPT:
    a. Reassure patient using quiet voice
    b. Encourage slow, normal breaths
    c. Administer O_2 as needed
    d. Remove any objects from patient's oral cavity

12 Ergonomics and Work-Related Musculoskeletal Disorders

COMPETENCIES

1. Apply ergonomic principles in dental hygiene practice, considering environmental, equipment, positioning, performance, and person-level factors.
2. Demonstrate strengthening and chairside stretching exercises. Also, discuss the importance of a regular exercise regimen.
3. Compare and contrast common **repetitive strain injuries (RSIs)** in terms of signs, symptoms, and risk factors. Also, practice chairside measures for prevention of RSIs and other musculoskeletal disorders (MSDs) that a dental hygienist should take before, during, and after patient care appointments.
4. Demonstrate exercises recommended for reducing the risk of injury.

SHORT ANSWER QUESTIONS

1. If the patient is in the supine position, about where should be the patient's mouth be in relation to the seated clinician?

_____

_____

_____

_____

2. Why is it not recommended for a right-handed clinician to work beyond the 8 o'clock position (4 o'clock for a left-handed clinician)?

_____

_____

_____

_____

3. List four benefits of an external fulcrum.

_____

_____

_____

_____

4. List five appointment control measures to implement within the daily dental hygiene schedule to reduce RSI.

_____

_____

_____

_____

_____

5. List three exercise regimes that will assist in reducing RSI.

_____

_____

_____

_____

6. List and briefly describe the five categories of motion.

_____

_____

_____

_____

_____

FILL IN THE BLANK STATEMENTS

Select the best term from the chapter and complete the following statements.

1. Environmental factors that impact musculoskeletal health in the practice of dental hygiene include _____ and _____.

2. Equipment factors that impact musculoskeletal health in the practice of dental hygiene include _____, _____ and _____.

3. When treating maxillary teeth, the maxillary plane should be _____ to the floor.

4. When treating mandibular teeth, the mandibular plane should be _____ to the floor.

5. Maintaining _____ of the wrist, elbow, arm, and shoulder is the best prevention for occupational pain.

6. _____ is caused by a compressed nerve in a narrow passageway on the palm side of the wrist.

MULTIPLE CHOICE QUESTIONS

Complete each question by circling the best answer.

1. A clinician's chair that positions the hygienist too high causes the spine, back, and shoulders to support the body weight. A clinician's chair that positions the hygienist too low causes the clinician to slump and sit with a curved spine.
   a. Both statements are true.
   b. Both statements are false.
   c. The first statement is true, the second statement is false.
   d. The first statement is false, the second statement is true.

2. The clinician's chair should allow the clinician's feet to be flat on the floor with knees positioned slightly below the hips. Knees should be a slight angle of 105-125° hip angle.
   a. Both statements are true.
   b. Both statements are false.
   c. The first statement is true, the second statement is false.
   d. The first statement is false, the second statement is true.

3. The most common patient position for treating most patient is:
   a. Upright
   b. Semi-upright
   c. Supine
   d. Trendelenburg

4. The most common patient position for patient education is:
   a. Upright
   b. Semi-upright
   c. Supine
   d. Trendelenburg

5. The most common patient position for treating a patient experiencing dizziness is:
   a. Upright
   b. Semi-upright
   c. Supine
   d. Trendelenburg

6. The most common patient position for treating patients with asthma is:
   a. Upright
   b. Semi-upright
   c. Supine
   d. Trendelenburg

7. The modified pen grasp includes all of the following characteristics EXCEPT:
   a. Using a four-finger grasp with the thumb
   b. A space between the index finger and thumb
   c. Firm grasp
   d. Light grasp

8. All of the following are characteristics of a fulcrum EXCEPT:
   a. Provides hand stabilization during instrumentation
   b. Reduces risk of RSI
   c. Fulcrum finger should be locked during activation
   d. Splitting middle finger and fulcrum finger increases instrument control

9. All of the following are symptoms of carpal tunnel syndrome EXCEPT:
   a. Numbness in the areas supplied by the median nerve
   b. Pain in hands
   c. Warm fingers
   d. Loss of strength in hands

10. RSI that is caused by compression of the brachial artery and plexus nerve trunk is:
    a. De Quervain's syndrome
    b. Lateral epicondylitis
    c. Cubital Tunnel syndrome
    d. Thoracic outlet compression

11. RSI that is caused by immobility of the shoulder because of severe shoulder injury or repeated occurrences of rotator cuff tendonitis is:
    a. Cubital tunnel syndrome
    b. Tension myalgia
    c. Cervical spondylolysis
    d. Adhesive capsulitis

12. RSI that affects the ulnar nerve as it crosses behind the elbow is:
    a. Guyon's canal syndrome
    b. Cubital tunnel syndrome
    c. De Quervain's syndrome
    d. Lateral epicondylitis

13. RSI that affects the radial nerve entrapped in the radial tunnel is:
    a. Radial tunnel syndrome
    b. Tension myalgia
    c. Cervical spondylolysis
    d. Adhesive capsulitis

14. RSI that is a degenerative elbow disorder resulting from inflammation of the wrist extensor tendons on the lateral epicondyle of the elbow is called:
    a. Rotator cuff injury
    b. Lateral epicondylitis
    c. Cervical spondylitis
    d. Cubital tunnel syndrome

15. All of the following are correct clinical positions EXCEPT:
    a. Shoulders parallel to the floor
    b. Neck centered with minimal bending <20 degrees in any direction
    c. Elbows relaxed and close to the body
    d. Wrists aligned with hand and forearm with flexion >15 degrees

CASE STUDY

Create a daily strengthening exercise plan to prevent RSI that includes adaptive movements for the workplace.

_____

_____

_____

_____

_____

_____

_____

_____

_____

_____

_____

_____

_____

_____

_____

13 Personal, Dental, and Health Histories

COMPETENCIES

1. Explain the purpose of recording personal, dental, and health histories.
2. Discuss a health history assessment, the data collection process, and documentation by utilizing patient-centered interviewing techniques.
3. Describe the legal and ethical issues related to collecting and documenting health history information.
4. Discuss the process of decision making after obtaining the health history to include the interpretation of patient data, understanding the indications and rationale for prophylactic antibiotic premedication, and identifying the need for collaboration with other health care professionals for medical risk assessment to establish an individual dental hygiene care plan.

SHORT ANSWER QUESTIONS

1. List reasons why collecting a patient's personal history is important.

_____

_____

_____

_____

2. List reasons why collecting a patient's medical history is important.

_____

_____

_____

3. What are the two ethical obligations dental hygienist should apply when communicating verbally and nonverbally to patients?

_____

_____

4. List reasons why the dental history of a patient is important.

_____

_____

_____

_____

_____

_____

_____

_____

5. List conditions that would initiate a medical consultation.

_____

_____

_____

_____

6. Reviewing Table 13-2, question 2, if your patient answered "yes" to feeling anxious during dental appointments, what follow-up questions would you ask?

_____

_____

_____

_____

7. Your patient notes several food, environmental, and medication allergies on his medical history form. What would be a major concern when treating this patient?

_____

_____

_____

_____

8. Your patient notes that she has epilepsy. Her last episode was a week ago. She reports that she has not taken her medication today. Can she be treated today? What other concerns do you have?

_____

_____

_____

_____

9. Your patient states that he has diabetes mellitus. His last HbA1c was 10. He admits that he is not diligent with his diet or his blood sugar testing. Does he need premedication? Medical consult? Can he be treated in your office today? What other concerns do you have?

_____

_____

_____

_____

FILL IN THE BLANK STATEMENTS

1. Patients that experience stress, fear, and anxiety during the dental visit may be at risk for a _____.

2. The primary reason for a patient seeking dental services is _____.

3. Prophylactic _____ is recommended for patients at risk of _____.

4. _____ requires all individually identifiable personal health information or health-related information be protected unless the written approval of the patient or patient's guardian is obtained.

5. One month following a myocardial infarction, _____ determines a level of recovery and risk to progress with dental procedures.

MULTIPLE CHOICE QUESTIONS

Complete each question by circling the best answer.

1. All of the following are reasons the dental hygienist collects personal, medical, and dental information EXCEPT:
   a. Develop clinician-patient rapport
   b. Provide clinician paternalism
   c. Determine the need for medical consult
   d. Minimize possible risks

2. One of the main reasons to conduct a patient's health history interview is to:
   a. Collect insurance information
   b. Form a rapport with the patient's physician
   c. Develop a clinician-patient partnership
   d. Screen for oral diseases

3. Applying motivational interviewing techniques during the interview process promotes better communication between patient and clinician. Change talk encourages patients to discuss their reasons and need for dental care.
   a. Both statements are true.
   b. Both statements are false.
   c. The first statement is true, the second statement is false.
   d. The first statement is false, the second statement is true.

4. Dental hygienists are responsible for mandatory reporting all of the following EXCEPT:
   a. Infectious diseases
   b. Domestic violence
   c. Abuse
   d. CDC breach

5. A patient with poorly controlled diabetes would have an ASA classification of:
   a. I
   b. II
   c. III
   d. IV

6. A patient who smokes tobacco would have an ASA classification of:
   a. I
   b. II
   c. III
   d. IV

7. While completing the health history interview, the patient states that her blood pressure runs high and she has a family history of cardiovascular disease. She has not seen a physician in over 5 years. What Human Needs Conceptual Model deficit does this reflect?
   a. Protection from Health Risks
   b. Freedom from Fear and Stress
   c. Conceptualization and Problem Solving
   d. Responsibility for Oral Health

8. Risk factors that may affect a patient's willingness or ability to seek adequate oral health care are considered:
   a. Health literacy
   b. Personal autonomy
   c. Social determinants of health
   d. Economic disparity

9. Your patient experienced a myocardial infarction 1 month ago. What must occur before treating this patient?
   a. The patient should be able to walk up a flight of stairs without limitations.
   b. The dental hygienist needs medical clearance from the patient's cardiologist before proceeding.
   c. The patient requires premedication prior to treatment.
   d. The patient should reschedule for 6 months later.

10. In general, which of the following conditions require premedication?
    a. Joint replacement
    b. Organ transplant
    c. Indwelling vascular catheter
    d. Prosthetic cardiac valve

11. Your patient states that he used cocaine the previous night. What is the contraindication of care for this patient?
    a. Vasoconstrictors in local anesthesia
    b. Nitrous oxide
    c. Ionizing radiation
    d. Ultrasonic instrumentation

12. Which is NOT a recommended prophylactic antibiotic premedication?
    a. Amoxicillin 2 g
    b. Clindamycin 2 g
    c. Cephalexin 2 g
    d. Azithromycin 500 mg

13. The patient's treatment record should include all of the following EXCEPT:
    a. Referrals
    b. Physician's contact information
    c. Dental insurance information
    d. Informed consent

Age	60	SCENARIO
Gender	M	
Height	5'10"	**EOE/IOE:**
Weight	240 lb	Herpetic lesion on vermillion border adjacent to tooth #9-10
B/P	160/98 mm Hg	Palpable submandibular lymph nodes
Chief Complaint	"my gums bleed when I brush" "my wife says I have bad breath"	**Periodontal Findings:** Generalized pocket depths of 5-7 mm, 1-2 mm recession Generalized moderate calculus, biofilm, bleeding Heavy stain
Medical History Current Medications	Asthma Hypertension Knee replacement 6 months ago High cholesterol Allergy to sulfa and penicillin 1) Albuterol inhaler prn 2) Breo inhaler qd 3) Singular 20 mg qd 4) Hydrochlorothiazide 50 mg qd 5) Lipitor 20 mg qd 6) Vitamin D 2000 IU qd	**Radiographic Findings:** Moderate bone loss generalized Caries on several interproximal surfaces **Dental Findings:** Several areas of decay, broken restorations, need for endo and crowns Has not seen a dental hygienist or dentist for over 5 years. He started a new job that offers dental insurance
Social History	6 oz of whiskey daily Smokes 1 pack of cigarettes a day Father died from heart attack age 58 Mother died of colon cancer age 55	Works as a customer service rep for a sporting equipment company

1. What follow-up questions would you ask your patient?
   a. high blood pressure?
   b. joint replacement?
      i. Name and number of surgeon
      ii. Recommended premed?
   c. Does he take is medications regularly?
   d. Last asthma attack?
      i. Hospitalization?

2. What is his ASA classification? Why?

   _____

   _____

   _____

3. Can you treat this patient today? Why or why not?

   _____

   _____

   _____

Age	40	SCENARIO
Gender	F	
Height	5'4"	**EOE/IOE:**
Weight	140 lb	Xerostomia
B/P	140/88 mm Hg	**Periodontal Findings:**
Chief Complaint	"I'm here for a routine cleaning" "I've noticed my front tooth is loose"	Generalized pocket depths of 3-5 mm, 1-2 mm recession, localized pocket depths 7-8 mm around #7 with class III mobility Generalized slight calculus, biofilm, moderate bleeding
Medical History	Type 1 Diabetes recent (HbA1c) was 9.8	**Radiographic Findings:**
Current Medications	insulin glargine 16 units hs (long-acting) before meals	Generalized slight bone loss posterior Severe bone loss #7, endo treated 5 years ago
Social History	4 oz wine occasionally Smokes marijuana daily	**Dental Findings:** Stable restorations

4. What follow-up questions would you ask your patient?

_____

_____

_____

_____

5. Is this patient controlled or uncontrolled?

_____

6. What services could you provide for her?
   a. In-office finger stick or referral for testing

7. What is her ASA classification? Why?

_____

_____

_____

8. Can you treat this patient today? Why or why not?

_____

_____

_____

_____

14 Vital Signs

1. Discuss vital signs and the importance of minimizing risk of a medical emergency via vital signs assessment.
2. Discuss the significance of body temperature, assess and record body temperature, and make decisions based on observed body temperature.
3. Discuss the significance of pulse rate, assess and record pulse rate, and make decisions based on observed pulse rate.
4. Discuss the significance of respiration rate, assess and record respiration rate, and make decisions based on observed respiration rate.
5. Discuss the significance of blood pressure, assess and record blood pressure, and make decisions based on observed blood pressure.

SHORT ANSWER QUESTIONS

1. List guidelines to assist clinician in obtaining accurate patient vital signs.

_____
_____
_____
_____
_____
_____
_____
_____

2. Narrow airways may cause obstructed breathing in what diseases?

_____
_____
_____
_____
_____
_____

3. What is the period of diminished or absent Korotkoff sounds during the manual measurement of blood pressure?

_____
_____
_____
_____
_____
_____

4. What factors influence pulse rate?

_____

_____

_____

_____

_____

_____

_____

_____

5. What factors influence blood pressure?

_____

_____

_____

_____

_____

_____

_____

_____

_____

_____

_____

_____

_____

_____

6. What is an acceptable range of oral temperature for adults?

_____

_____

_____

7. What is an acceptable pulse range for adults?

_____

_____

_____

8. What is an acceptable range of respirations for adults?

_____

_____

_____

9. What is an acceptable blood pressure range for adults?

_____

_____

_____

FILL IN THE BLANK STATEMENTS

Select the best term from the chapter and complete the following statements.

1. An abnormally elevated heart rate of more than 100 beats per minute is called _____.

2. An abnormally slow heart rate of less than 60 beats per minute is called _____.

3. _____ is rapid breathing greater than 20 respirations per minute.

4. Rhythmic knocking sounds heard when measuring blood pressure using a stethoscope are called _____.

MULTIPLE CHOICE QUESTIONS

Complete each question by circling the best answer.

1. The techniques for assessing vital signs are all of the following EXCEPT:
   a. Auscultation
   b. Percussion
   c. Palpation
   d. Visual inspection

2. Systolic blood pressure measures the maximum pressure occurring in the blood vessels during cardiac ventricular contraction. Diastolic blood pressure measures the minimum pressure occurring against the arterial walls as a result of cardiac ventricular relaxation.
   a. Both statements are true.
   b. Both statements are false.
   c. The first statement is true, the second statement is false.
   d. The first statement is false, the second statement is true.

3. Which of the following area of the brain is responsible for body temperature regulation?
   a. Hippocampus
   b. Thalamus
   c. Hypothalamus
   d. Hippothalamus

4. Disposable thermometers are typically used for oral screenings. Mercury-in-glass thermometers are the standard of care for dental chairside use.
   a. Both statements are true.
   b. Both statements are false.
   c. The first statement is true, the second statement is false.
   d. The first statement is false, the second statement is true.

5. Pulsus alternas may be an indication of:
   a. Premature ventricular contractions
   b. Atrial failure
   c. Cardiac arrest
   d. Ventricular failure

6. A systolic blood pressure reading above 180 mm Hg is a:
   a. Normal reading
   b. Hypertensive crisis
   c. Hypotension
   d. Requires premedication

7. Which finger(s) should the clinician use when determining a patient's radial pulse?
   a. Thumb and index finger
   b. Thumb and middle finger
   c. Index finger
   d. Middle and index finger

CASE STUDY MS. FERRARA

Age	79	SCENARIO
Gender	female	**EOE/IOE:**
Height	5'4"	Generalized slight biofilm, generalized moderate calculus mandibular anterior, generalized moderate extrinsic brown stain
Weight	130 lb	
B/P	180/110 mm Hg taken twice with no change	
Chief Complaint	Routine cleaning, notices some bleeding maxillary right	#2-4 interproximally moderate/heavy calculus subgingivally
Medical History	Depression High blood pressure Reflux Asthma	**Periodontal Findings:** Probe readings 2-4 mm generalized with 1-2 mm recession generalized Slight BOP generalized Generalized moderate gingival inflammation
Current Medications	Singular Albuterol inhaler Breo inhaler Lasix Fluoxetine Bystolic Oscimin	#2-4 have 6 mm interproximal bleeding **Radiographic Findings:** #30 requires a crown
Social History	Non-drinker Non-smoker	**Dental Findings:** Caries on #28

Using the data from this patient, develop a Human Needs Conceptual model for treatment.

Dental Hygiene Diagnosis (unmet human need)	Etiology (due to…)	Signs and Symptoms (evidenced by…)	Patient Goals (expected outcomes)
Protection from Health Risks			
Freedom from Fear and Stress			
Freedom from Pain			
Wholesome Facial Image			
Skin and Mucous Membrane Integrity of the Head and Neck			
Biologically Sound and Functional Dentition			
Conceptualization and Problem Solving			
Responsibility for Oral Health			

COMPETENCY 14-1 MEASURING THE RADIAL PULSE

Objective

Student will accurately take and record patient's pulse by following stated procedure and protocol.

Evaluation and Grading Criteria

Instructor will assign grades for each performance criteria.

<u>3</u> Student competently met stated criteria
<u>2</u> Student required minimal assistance to meet criteria
<u>1</u> Student showed uncertainty when attempting criteria
<u>0</u> Student was not prepared and needs to repeat criteria
N/A Student was not evaluated

Performance Standards

Instructor shall identify steps that are critical with an asterisk (*)

Performance Criteria	*	Self	Peer	Instructor	Comments
Equipment: ■ Wristwatch with a second hand ■ Pen ■ Patient record ■ Vital signs chart					
STEPS 1. Use a wristwatch with a second hand.					
2. Perform hand hygiene.					
3. Explain purpose and method of procedure to the patient. Advise patient to relax and not to speak.					
4. Have patient assume a sitting position, bend the patient's elbow 90 degrees, and support the patient's lower arm on the armrest of the chair. Extend the wrist with the palm up.					
5. Place first two fingers of hand along the patient's radial artery (thumb side of wrist) and lightly compress.					
6. Obliterate the pulse initially, then relax pressure so that the pulse is easily palpable.					
7. Determine rhythm and quality of the pulse (regular, regularly irregular, full and strong, weak and thready).					
8. When pulse can be felt regularly, use the watch's second hand and begin to count the rate, starting with 0 and then 1, and so on.					
9. If the pulse is regular, count for 30 seconds and multiply the total by 2.					
10. If the pulse is irregular, count for a full minute.					

Continued

Performance Criteria	*	Self	Peer	Instructor	Comments
11. Record heart rate (beats per minute [BPM]), rhythm of the heart (regular or irregular), the quality of the pulse (thready, strong, weak, bounding), and the date in the chart. Pulse rates outside the normal range should be evaluated by the patient's physician.					
12. Document completion of this service in the patient's record under "Services Rendered." Record heart rate (BPM), rhythm of the heart (regular, regularly irregular, or irregularly irregular), the quality of the pulse (thready and weak [not easily felt], strong and full [easily felt]), and the date in the record.					
ADDITIONAL COMMENTS					

COMPETENCY 14-2 RESPIRATION

Objective
Student will accurately take and record patient's respiration by following stated procedure and protocol.

Evaluation and Grading Criteria
Instructor will assign grades for each performance criteria.

3 Student competently met stated criteria
2 Student required minimal assistance to meet criteria
1 Student showed uncertainty when attempting criteria
0 Student was not prepared and needs to repeat criteria
N/A Student was not evaluated

Performance Standards
Instructor shall identify steps that are critical with an asterisk (*)

Performance Criteria	*	Self	Peer	Instructor	Comments
Equipment ■ Wristwatch with a second hand ■ Pen ■ Patient record ■ Vital signs chart					
STEPS 1. Use a wristwatch with a second hand.					
2. Place hand along the patient's radial artery and inconspicuously observe the patient's chest before or after taking the patient's pulse rate.					
3. Observe the rise and fall of patient's chest. Count complete respiratory cycles (one inspiration and one expiration).					
4. For an adult, count the number of respirations in 30 seconds and multiply that number by 2. For a young child, count respirations for a full minute.					
5. If an adult has respirations with an irregular rhythm, or if respirations are abnormally slow or fast (<12 or >20 breaths/minute), count for a full minute.					
6. While counting, note whether depth is shallow, normal, or deep and whether rhythm is normal or one of the altered patterns.					
7. Document in the patient record the completion of this service in the patient's record under "Services Rendered."					
ADDITIONAL COMMENTS					

COMPETENCY 14-3 ASSESSING BLOOD PRESSURE BY AUSCULTATION

Objective

Student will accurately take and record patient's blood pressure by following stated procedure and protocol.

Evaluation and Grading Criteria

Instructor will assign grades for each performance criteria.

    3 Student competently met stated criteria
    2 Student required minimal assistance to meet criteria
    1 Student showed uncertainty when attempting criteria
    0 Student was not prepared and needs to repeat criteria
N/A Student was not evaluated

Performance Standards

Instructor shall identify steps that are critical with an asterisk (*)

Performance Criteria	*	Self	Peer	Instructor	Comments
Gather equipment: ■ Blood pressure cuff or sphygmomanometer ■ Stethoscope ■ Pen ■ Patient record ■ Vital signs chart					
STEPS 1. Allow patient to sit quietly for at least 5 minutes with back and feet supported (legs uncrossed).					
2. Ask patient about recent activities that could alter the patient's normal blood pressure. Avoid assessing blood pressure if patient has ingested caffeine, smoked or used other nicotine products, or exercised within 30 minutes.					
3. Determine proper cuff size. Inspect the parts of the release valve and the pressure bulb. The valve should be clean and freely movable in either direction.					
4. Perform hand hygiene.					
5. Explain purpose of the procedure but avoid talking to patient for at least a minute before taking the patient's blood pressure.					
6. Assist patient to a comfortable sitting position, with arm slightly flexed, forearm supported and at heart level.					
7. Expose the upper arm fully.					
8. Palpate brachial artery. Position the cuff approximately 1 inch above the antecubital space.					
9. Center arrows marked on the cuff over the brachial artery.					

Continued

Performance Criteria	*	Self	Peer	Instructor	Comments
10. Be sure cuff is fully deflated. Wrap cuff evenly and snugly around the upper arm. Center arrow on cuff over artery. If there is no arrow, estimate center of bladder and place over artery.					
11. Be sure manometer is positioned for easy reading.					
12. If patient's normal systolic pressure is unknown, palpate the radial artery and rapidly inflate cuff to a pressure 30 mm Hg above the point at which radial pulsation disappears. Deflate the cuff quickly and wait 30 seconds.					
13. Place stethoscope earpieces in ears and be sure sounds are clear, not muffled.					
14. Place diaphragm (or the bell) of the stethoscope over the brachial artery in the antecubital fossa. The antecubital fossa is the depression in the underside of the arm at the bend of the elbow. Avoid contact with blood pressure cuff or clothing.					
15. Close valve of pressure bulb clockwise until tight.					
16. Inflate cuff to 30 mm Hg above patient's normal systolic level.					
17. Slowly release valve, allowing the needle of the aneroid gauge to fall at a rate of 2 mm Hg per second.					
18. Note point on manometer at which the first clear sound is heard.					
19. Continue cuff deflation, noting point on the manometer at which the sound muffles (phase IV) and disappears (phase V). Listen for 10 to 20 mm Hg after last sound.					
20. Deflate cuff rapidly. To determine an average blood pressure and ensure a correct reading, wait 2 minutes, then repeat procedure for the same arm. Calculate the average of the two readings.					
21. Remove cuff from patient's arm. Assist patient to a comfortable position and cover upper arm.					
22. Disinfect earpieces of stethoscope and fold cuff, and store properly in a cool, dry place.					
23. Discuss findings with patient.					
24. Document completion of this service in patient's record under "Services Rendered." Record in patient's record the systolic over the diastolic blood pressure reading in mm Hg, the date, cuff size if it was an atypical size, and arm used for measurement					

Performance Criteria	*	Self	Peer	Instructor	Comments
25. Prevention of Disease Transmission * Critical error 5 points deduction					
ADDITIONAL COMMENTS					

15 Pharmacologic History

OBJECTIVES/COMPETENCIES

1. Discuss the importance of formulating and interpreting a comprehensive pharmacologic history.
2. Identify fundamental questions to gather a comprehensive pharmacologic history, and do the following:
   - Describe adverse drug events, including side effects, drug toxicity, and drug hypersensitivity reactions.
   - Describe common side effects caused by medications.
   - Discuss strategies to improve patient compliance with medication use.
     a. Discuss dental hygiene interventions to manage the oral complications of medication use.

SHORT ANSWER QUESTIONS

1. Which education technique helps ensure a patient's understanding of using a medication correctly?

_____

_____

2. List the reasons why a patient may take a medication.

_____

_____

_____

_____

_____

_____

_____

3. List the eight assessment questions to why a medication is prescribed.

_____

_____

_____

_____

_____

_____

_____

_____

_____

_____

_____

_____

_____

_____

_____

_____

4. What oral medicament is recommended for a patient with hyposalivation?

_____

_____

5. Identify pharmaceutical recommendations for the treatment of xerostomia.

_____

_____

_____

_____

_____

_____

FILL IN THE BLANK STATEMENTS

Select the best term from the chapter and complete the following statements.

1. _____ is when a drug is not used as intended or prescribed.

2. Medications that are concerned with target tissues to produce a desired change are known as the _____.

3. Medications that produce an undesired change are known as _____.

4. Medications that cause toxin-induced cell damage and cell death are known as _____.

5. Medications or their metabolites that trigger an immune response are known as _____.

6. Medications that cause negative effects on fetal development are known as _____.

7. The drug classification that stimulates serous salivary flow is _____.

MULTIPLE CHOICE QUESTIONS

Complete each question by circling the best answer.

1. The dose schedule for an adult includes all of the following EXCEPT:
   a. Name of medication
   b. Frequency
   c. Measured quantity
   d. Cost of medication

2. The dental hygienist should create a written take-home record of each patient's medications list, including dose schedules and the name of the prescribing physician, as mandated by law. This written record is helpful to all health professionals treating the patient and may be especially useful during an emergency situation.
   a. Both statements are true.
   b. Both statements are false.
   c. The first statement is true, the second statement is false.
   d. The first statement is false, the second statement is true.

3. All of the following drug classifications have the side effect of creating gingival enlargement EXCEPT:
   a. Cholinergics
   b. Calcium channel blockers
   c. Anticonvulsants
   d. Antirejection drugs

4. The patient medication list should be updated every year. Patient drug allergies should be recorded at the initial appointment only.
   a. Both statements are true.
   b. Both statements are false.
   c. The first statement is true, the second statement is false.
   d. The first statement is false, the second statement is true.

5. Children absorb medications faster than adults because of:
   a. Increased skin and mucous membrane permeability
   b. Immature adrenal glands
   c. Teratogenicity
   d. Underdeveloped liver

6. All of the following are true concerning medication doses for the elderly EXCEPT:
   a. Increased stomach acidity alters drug absorption rate
   b. Decreased liver and kidney function
   c. Double normal adult drug dosage
   d. Reduction of plasma proteins

7. All medications have the potential to cause adverse side effects. Medication interactions are rarely life threatening.
   a. Both statements are true.
   b. Both statements are false.
   c. The first statement is true, the second statement is false.
   d. The first statement is false, the second statement is true.

8. The government agency that is responsible for adopting the labeled risk for Pregnancy and Lactation Labeling Rule is
   a. CDC
   b. FDA
   c. NIH
   d. ADA

9. An undocumented or unexpected genetically linked side effect of a medication is a drug:
   a. Tolerance
   b. Hypersensitivity
   c. Idiosyncrasy
   d. Toxicity

10. All of the following may have adverse effects when taken with prescribed medications EXCEPT:
    a. Alcohol
    b. OTC supplements
    c. Certain foods
    d. Tobacco

11. Rapid drug metabolism causing the need to take larger doses of the drug to produce the same response is drug:
    a. Tolerance
    b. Hypersensitivity
    c. Idiosyncrasy
    d. Toxicity

12. A patient's medication management is influenced by all of the following EXCEPT:
    a. Lack of knowledge concerning mixing medications
    b. Lack of understanding concerning medication instructions
    c. Availability of non-prescription medications
    d. Over-the-counter medications and supplements

13. The negative effects that can occur when two or more drugs are taken together is a drug:
    a. Tolerance
    b. Hypersensitivity
    c. Interaction
    d. Toxicity

14. How a medication is absorbed, utilized, metabolized, and excreted from the body is called:
    a. Tolerance
    b. Hypersensitivity
    c. Interaction
    d. Pharmacokinetics

15. Your 25-year-old healthy female patient reports taking 81 mg of aspirin daily. She also reports no other health conditions. She states she saw an advertisement on the internet about the benefits of taking a baby aspirin daily to prevent a stroke. You find no evidence or family history of heart disease or a medical reason to take aspirin. Educating your patient on aspirin use and directing her to discuss this with her primary care physician would address what Human Needs Model deficit?
    a. Protection from Health Risks
    b. Freedom from Fear and Stress
    c. Conceptualization and Problem Solving
    d. Responsibility for Oral Health

16. Adverse negative effects of a drug during fetal development is:
    a. Teratogenicity
    b. Idiosyncrasy
    c. Hypersensitivity
    d. Pharmacokinetics

CASE STUDY: MR. ROSS

Age	78	**SCENARIO**
Gender	male	
Height	6'3"	**EOE/IOE:**
Weight	200 lb	Gingival stomatitis present on palate
B/P	125/70 mm Hg	Fissured tongue
Chief Complaint	Gingival tissues inflamed, having trouble eating	**Periodontal Findings:** Type III periodontal disease with severe gingivitis, generalized heavy biofilm, 2-3 mm recession generalized, missing molars on the right side, slight calculus generalized
Medical History	Stroke 5 years ago, left side paralyzed High cholesterol High blood pressure Depression Recent bed sore infection on left buttock and left heel Recent INR 3.5 Has a caregiver to assist his wife during the week	**Radiographic Findings:** No caries, no new periodontal findings **Dental Findings:** Maxillary partial denture needs adjustment
Current Medications	Warafin 10 mg once a day Lipitor 20 mg twice a day Prozac 20 mg twice a day Norvasc 10 mg twice a day Erythromycin 250 mg four times a day Not all medications are prescribed by the same physician	Wife reports serving healthy meals that include grapefruit and oatmeal for breakfast, leafy greens, and lunch and dinner with lean meats. Patient states he has difficulty and pain when chewing and his palate is sore. He also reports nausea and reflux.
Social History	Previous smoker Previous social drinker	

1. Investigate the current medications list.
   a. Are there any discrepancies or contraindications in doses/medications?

_____

_____

_____

_____

_____

_____

_____

2. Assist Mrs. Ross in developing a Medication Map.

_____
_____
_____
_____
_____
_____

3. Review current diet and counsel Mrs. Ross/caregiver on foods that may interfere with drug actions.

_____
_____
_____
_____
_____
_____

4. Is a consultation with his primary care physician warranted? Why or why not?

_____
_____
_____
_____
_____
_____
_____
_____
_____
_____

5. What is your first issue to address?

_____

_____

_____

6. Develop a dental hygiene care plan for Mr. Ross.

_____

_____

_____

_____

_____

_____

_____

_____

_____

_____

_____

_____

16 Assessment of Head and Neck Examination

SHORT ANSWER QUESTIONS

1. What is the condition in which lymph nodes are palpable and enlarged?

_____

_____

2. Where do the submandibular lymph nodes empty into?

_____

_____

3. What is located lingually between the maxillary central incisors?

_____

_____

4. Is the laryngopharynx visible during the intraoral clinical assessment?

_____

_____

5. Where do over 75% of head and neck cancers originate?

_____

_____

6. What is the surgical removal of a section of tissue for the purpose of diagnosis, to estimate prognosis, and to monitor the cause of disease?

   _____

   _____

7. Examining sample cells that are collected by scraping the surface of a lesion is considered what type of science?

   _____

   _____

8. Using a specially designed brush to remove sample cells from lesions that are atypical in appearance is considered what type of science?

   _____

   _____

9. Distinguishing a condition or disease from others that may manifest similar clinical signs or symptoms is considered what type of diagnosis?

   _____

   _____

10. Explain and demonstrate the differences between digital palpation, bidigital palpation, manual palpation, bimanual palpation, bilateral palpation, and circular compression.

    _____

    _____

    _____

    _____

    _____

    _____

    _____

    _____

VIDEO REVIEW QUESTIONS

The following questions are directed toward the extra- and intraoral videos located on Evolve. Watch the following videos before answering the questions:

- *Conducting Extraoral Assessments*
- *Conducting Intraoral Assessments*
- *Conducting an Oral CDx Brush Biopsy*

1. What is the clinician assessing during initial clinical inspection and before any palpation?

_____

_____

_____

_____

_____

_____

_____

2. What technique is used to palpate occipital nodes?

_____

_____

3. A patient's lack of facial expression may be an indication of what?

_____

_____

4. Which gland is adjacent to the masseter muscle during palpation?

_____

_____

5. What type of palpation is used when assessing superficial cervical nodes?

_____

_____

6. When rolling the tissue over each side of the angle of the mandible, what three glands are palpated?

_____

_____

_____

_____

_____

_____

7. Why does the clinician have the patient swallow during assessment?

_____

_____

_____

8. What type of palpation is used when examining the lower lip?

_____

_____

_____

9. What intraoral structure is observed when gently retracting the lower lip ?

_____

_____

_____

10. Which duct is being palpated at mark 1:33 in the *Conducting Intraoral Assessments* video?

_____

_____

_____

11. What type of palpation is used to inspect the retromolar pads and maxillary tuberosities?

_____

_____

_____

12. What patient movement assists the clinician in evaluating the palate and pharynx?

_____

_____

_____

13. Why is circular compression not recommended when palpating the soft palate?

_____

_____

_____

14. Which duct is being palpated in *Conducting Intraoral Assessments* video mark 4:40?

_____

_____

_____

_____

FILL IN THE BLANK STATEMENTS

1. Patient assessment begins with _____.

2. The four assessment skills utilized by the dental hygienist in patient clinical assessment are:

   a. _____

   b. _____

   c. _____

   d. _____

3. An _____ finding of the head region extraoral clinical assessment would be an eyebrow

   piercing while an _____ finding would be swelling and bruising around the eye.

4. An _____ finding of the neck region extraoral clinical assessment would be conspic-

   uous thyroid cartilage while an _____ finding would be an enlarged thyroid gland.

5. Deep cervical nodes drain the:

   a. _____

   b. _____

   c. _____

   d. _____

   e. _____

   f. _____

   g. _____

6. _____ Findings posterior to the most distal maxillary tooth are called the

   _____ while findings posterior to the most distal mandibular tooth are called the _____

   _____.

7. The four types of papilla located on the tongue are:

   a. _____

   b. _____

   c. _____

   d. _____

8. When describing an oral lesion, list the specific descriptive terms used for documentation.

   a. _____

   b. _____

   c. _____

   d. _____

   e. _____

   f. _____

   g. _____

82

Chapter **16** **Assessment of Head and Neck Examination**

9. List four risk factors for oropharyngeal cancer.
   a. _____

   b. _____

   c. _____

   d. _____

MULTIPLE CHOICE QUESTIONS

1. A flat, non-palpable lesion less than 1 cm is:
   a. Bulla
   b. Papule
   c. Macule
   d. Nodule

2. A raised fluid filled lesion less than 0.5 cm is:
   a. Ulcer
   b. Vesicle
   c. Pustule
   d. Bulla

3. A lesion that has lost the epithelial tissue layer and varies with size is:
   a. Pustule
   b. Vesicle
   c. Plaque
   d. Ulcer

4. A lesion surface that exhibits ridges and irregularities would be described as:
   a. Corrugated
   b. Fissured
   c. Cratered
   d. Verrucous

5. A lesion surface that exhibits a wrinkled appearance would be described as:
   a. Corrugated
   b. Indurated
   c. Cratered
   d. Crusted

6. A lesion consistency that contains calcified material would be described as:
   a. Hard
   b. Soft
   c. Rubbery
   d. Cemented

7. A lesion consistency that is moveable upon palpation with little or no fibrous or calcified tissue would be described as:
   a. Hard
   b. Soft
   c. Rubbery
   d. Cemented

8. The most common skin cancers are:
   a. Basal cell and squamous cell
   b. Oropharyngeal and basal cell
   c. Melanoma and squamous cell
   d. Melanoma and oropharyngeal

9. A lesion that measures 2-4 cm but without spread to lymph nodes or metastasis is categorized as stage:
   a. I
   b. II
   c. III
   d. IV

10. An abnormal mass of tissue that forms when cells grow and divide more than usual or when the mass of tissue never dies off is:
    a. Bulla
    b. Malignancy
    c. Neoplasm
    d. Nodule

11. A lesion that is located on either the right side or the left side is described as:
    a. Unilateral
    b. Bilateral
    c. Contralateral
    d. Ipsilateral

12. A lesion that is located on the opposite side from a specific structure is described as:
    a. Unilateral
    b. Bilateral
    c. Contralateral
    d. Ipsilateral

13. A lesion that is located on the same side as a specific structure is described as:
    a. Unilateral
    b. Bilateral
    c. Contralateral
    d. Ipsilateral

14. Which condition is directly related to increased cases of oropharyngeal cancer?
    a. HIV
    b. Hepatitis C
    c. HPV
    d. Smoking and tobacco use

Your 50-year-old patient reports for his routine maintenance appointment. He is a heavy alcohol user and reports smoking cigars once a month. He is retired and golfs several times a week. You notice a 4-mm lesion on the lateral surface of his tongue with erythroplakia.

1. What further questions do you ask your patient?
2. What diagnostic tests do you conduct?
3. What other data do you collect?
4. What education plan do you discuss with him?

_____

_____

_____

_____

_____

_____

_____

_____

_____

_____

_____

Performance Objective

By following a routine procedure that meets the stated protocols, the student will demonstrate the appropriate technique for **16-1 Conducting Extraoral Clinical Assessments: Head Regions**

Evaluation and Grading Criteria

Instructor will assign grades for each performance criteria.

<u>3</u> Student competently met stated criteria
<u>2</u> Student required minimal assistance to meet criteria
<u>1</u> Student showed uncertainty when attempting criteria
<u>0</u> Student was not prepared and needs to repeat criteria
<u>N/A</u> Student was not evaluated

Performance Standards

Instructor shall identify steps that are critical with an asterisk (*)

Performance Criteria	*	Self	Peer	Instructor	Comments
Equipment 1. Personal protective equipment 2. Hand mirror					
Extraoral Head Regions 1. Visually observe symmetry and coloration of face and neck with patient sitting upright. Allow patient to observe steps in a hand mirror for self-examination					
2. Visually inspect and bilaterally palpate forehead including frontal sinuses					
3. Visually inspect entire scalp by moving hair, especially around hairline, starting from one ear and proceeding to other ear; have patient lean head forward, and bilaterally palpate occipital nodes on each side of base of head					
4. Visually inspect and bilaterally palpate external ear, as well as scalp, face, and auricular nodes around each ear					
5. Visually inspect eyes with their movements and responses to light and action					
6. Visually inspect and bilaterally palpate external nose, starting at the root of nose and proceeding to its apex					
7. Visually inspect inferior to orbits, noting use of muscles of facial expression; visually inspect and bilaterally palpate each side of face and facial nodes, moving from infraorbital region to labial commissure and then to surface of the mandible; visually inspect and bilaterally palpate maxillary sinuses. Ask patient to open and close mouth several times; then ask patient to move opened jaw left, then right, and then forward; ask if there is pain or tenderness experienced and note sounds made by either joint. To further access TMJs, gently place finger into outer part of each external acoustic meatus during these movements					

Continued

Performance Criteria	*	Self	Peer	Instructor	Comments
8. Visually inspect and bilaterally palpate masseter and parotid by starting in front of each ear, moving to zygomatic arch and inferior to angle of the mandible; then place fingers of each hand over masseter muscle and ask patient to clench teeth together several times					
9. Visually inspect and bilaterally palpate chin					
10. Documentation	*				
11. Prevention of Disease Transmission	*				
ADDITIONAL COMMENTS					

Performance Objective

By following a routine procedure that meets the stated protocols, the student will demonstrate the appropriate technique for **16-2 Conducting Extraoral Clinical Assessments: Neck Regions**

Evaluation and Grading Criteria

Instructor will assign grades for each performance criteria.

3 Student competently met stated criteria
2 Student required minimal assistance to meet criteria
1 Student showed uncertainty when attempting criteria
0 Student was not prepared and needs to repeat criteria
N/A Student was not evaluated

Performance Standards

Instructor shall identify steps that are critical with an asterisk (*)

Performance Criteria	*	Self	Peer	Instructor	Comments
Equipment 3. Personal protective equipment 4. Hand mirror					
Neck Regions 12. Have patient lower chin and manually palpate submandibular and sublingual glands as well as the associated nodes directly underneath chin and on inferior border of mandible; then push the tissue in area over bony inferior border of mandible on each side, where it is grasped and rolled					
13. With patient looking straight ahead, manually palpate with two hands on each side of neck superficial cervical nodes, starting inferior to ear and continuing length of SCMs surface to the clavicles; then, have patient tilt head to each side to palpate superior deep cervical nodes on underside of anterior and posterior aspects of SCMs. Then, have the patient raise shoulders up and forward to palpate over each trapezius muscle surface inferior deep cervical, accessory, and supraclavicular nodes					
14. Locate thyroid cartilage and pass fingers up and down thyroid gland, examining for abnormal masses and overall size; then, place one hand on each side of trachea and gently displace thyroid gland tissue to contralateral side of neck while other hand manually palpates the displaced tissue. Compare two lobes of thyroid for size and texture using visual inspection and bimanual palpation. Ask patient to swallow to check for gland mobility by visually inspecting it while it moves superiorly and inferiorly; patient may need water to swallow. Finally, bidigitally palpate both hyoid bone and larynx and deliberately move each one gently					

Continued

Performance Criteria	*	Self	Peer	Instructor	Comments
15. Documentation	*				
16. Prevention of Disease Transmission	*				
ADDITIONAL COMMENTS					

17 Hard Tissue Assessment and Dental Charting

COMPETENCIES

1. Apply the proper methods of documentation required to fulfill dental hygiene responsibilities.
2. Demonstrate the use of different tooth-numbering systems and proper application of charting symbols.
3. Discuss the classification of dental caries and restorations.
4. Recognize hard tissue assessment methods including identification of signs and symptoms of dental caries, tooth damage, and clinically evident developmental anomalies.
5. Compare different malocclusion classifications.
6. Discuss common problems of occlusion.
7. Integrate tooth assessment and documentation into the dental hygiene process of care.

SHORT ANSWER QUESTIONS

1. What phase(s) of the dental hygiene process of care include(s) the initial hard tissue exam?

   _____

   _____

2. What phase(s) of the dental hygiene process of care include(s) hard tissue exam and updates?

   _____

   _____

3. What are the three goals of the hard tissue exam?

   _____

   _____

   _____

   _____

   _____

4. What does nomenclature DAQT stand for?

   _____

   _____

5. List the sites that are prone to caries.

   _____

   _____

   _____

   _____

   _____

   _____

6. List and briefly describe the types of dental caries.

_____

_____

_____

_____

_____

_____

_____

_____

_____

_____

_____

_____

_____

_____

_____

_____

_____

7. List and briefly describe caries by location.

_____

_____

_____

_____

_____

_____

_____

_____

_____

_____

_____

_____

_____

_____

_____

_____

8. What is the deviation from normal relationship between maxilla and mandible while in centric occlusion?

_____

_____

9. What is the ideal molar relationship when the primary teeth are in centric occlusion?

_____

_____

10. Describe a mesial step in primary centric occlusion.

_____

_____

_____

11. Describe a distal step in primary centric occlusion.

_____

_____

_____

12. List several parafunctional habits.

_____

_____

_____

_____

13. List the five approaches in assessing dental caries.

_____

_____

_____

_____

_____

14. List and briefly define the types of dental caries.

_____

_____

_____

_____

_____

_____

FILL IN THE BLANK STATEMENTS

Select the best term from the chapter and complete the following statements.

1. The exact location and condition of teeth are documented in a(n) _____.

2. _____ allow for identifying and charting individual teeth.

3. Contact relationship between maxilla and mandible in a closed position is referred to as _____.

4. Equal distribution of force when most maxillary and mandibular teeth touch is referred to as _____.

5. _____ is a system to evaluate occlusion.

6. The primary maxillary canine that occludes with the distal half of the mandibular canine is considered _____.

7. Movement of the mandible outside of normal performance is considered _____.

Complete each question by circling the best answer.

1. All of the following describe the uses of a hard tissue exam EXCEPT:
   a. Describes current patient dental health status
   b. Allows for concise communication with all that are involved in patient care
   c. Is the main resource to mass casualty victim identification
   d. Is a legal document of care that is provided

2. Quadrants in adult dentition include three anterior teeth and five posterior teeth. Sextants in adult dentition are divided into anterior and posterior sections.
   a. Both statements are true.
   b. Both statements are false.
   c. The first statement is true, the second statement is false.
   d. The first statement is false, the second statement is true.

3. Applying the Universal Numbering System, the permanent maxillary left first molar is expressed as what tooth number?
   a. 3
   b. 14
   c. 15
   d. 19

4. Applying the Universal Numbering System, identify nomenclature of tooth number 30.
   a. Permanent maxillary left second molar
   b. Permanent mandibular left first molar
   c. Permanent mandibular right first molar
   d. Permanent mandibular left second molar

5. What is the tooth-numbering system that uses two digits to identify each tooth whereby the first number indicates the quadrant and the second number indicates the specific tooth?
   a. Universal Numbering System
   b. International Numbering system
   c. Black's Classification System
   d. Palmer's Notation Method

6. The most common type of acquired tooth damage is:
   a. Fracture
   b. Attrition
   c. Caries
   d. Abrasion

7. Evaluating for caries using the explorer assessment method is not recommended because it interferes with the tooth's ability to remineralize. The explorer assessment method of caries detection may inoculate otherwise heathy tooth structure with pathogenic bacteria such as *Treponema denticola*.
   a. Both statements are true.
   b. Both statements are false.
   c. The first statement is true, the second statement is false.
   d. The first statement is false, the second statement is true.

8. Overjet is the term used to describe the horizontal protrusion when teeth meet in centric occlusion. Overbite is the term used to describe vertical overlap when teeth meet in centric occlusion.
   a. Both statements are true.
   b. Both statements are false.
   c. The first statement is true, the second statement is false.
   d. The first statement is false, the second statement is true.

9. In a normal molar relationship, the mesiobuccal cusp of the maxillary permanent first molar occludes with the mesiobuccal groove of the mandibular permanent first molar. In a normal canine relationship, the maxillary permanent canine occludes with the distal half of the mandibular permanent canine and the mesial half of the mandibular first premolar.
   a. Both statements are true.
   b. Both statements are false.
   c. The first statement is true, the second statement is false.
   d. The first statement is false, the second statement is true.

10. An occlusion classification in which the maxillary and mandibular anterior teeth meet at the incisal edged in centric occlusion is:
    a. End-to-end
    b. Edge-to-edge
    c. Crossbite
    d. Normal occlusion

11. An occlusion classification in which the maxillary teeth are positioned lingual to the mandibular teeth is:
    a. End-to-end
    b. Edge-to-edge
    c. Crossbite
    d. Normal occlusion

12. An occlusion classification in which the mesiobuccal cusp of the permanent maxillary first molar is positioned distal to the mesial buccal groove of the permanent mandibular first molar by at least the width of a premolar, whereas the maxillary permanent canine is distal to the distal surface of the mandibular permanent canine by at least the width of a premolar, is:
    a. Class I malocclusion
    b. Class II malocclusion
    c. Class III malocclusion
    d. Class IV malocclusion

13. An occlusion classification in which teeth are not preferably aligned despite normal canine and molar occlusion is:
    a. Class I malocclusion
    b. Class II malocclusion
    c. Class III malocclusion
    d. Class IV malocclusion

14. Misshapen small, supernumerary teeth are:
    a. Mesiodens
    b. Hypodontia
    c. Hyperdontia
    d. Dens a dente

15. Abnormal distortion of a tooth caused by trauma during tooth development is:
    a. Hypodontia
    b. Fusion
    c. Germination
    d. Dilacerations

16. The absence of one or more teeth is:
    a. Mesiodens
    b. Hypodontia
    c. Germination
    d. Microdontia

17. Autosomal dominant, autosomal recessive, or X-linked genetic disturbance of enamel development is:
    a. Hutchinson's incisors
    b. Microdontia
    c. Amelogenesis imperfecta
    d. Mulberry molar

18. An autosomal dominant inheritance pattern characterized by teeth with normal crowns and abnormal roots related to defect in Hertwig's epithelial root sheath is:
    a. Type I dentin dysplasia
    b. Type II dentin dysplasia
    c. Dentinogenesis imperfecta
    d. Amenogenesis imperfecta

19. An anomaly in which the crowns of teeth develop normally but the pulp chambers are enlarged is:
    a. Macrodontia
    b. Taurodontism
    c. Hyperdontia
    d. Mesiodens

20. A 20-year-old female patient presents with rampant caries. What Human Needs Conceptual model deficits does this address?
    a. Wholesome Facial Image
    b. Skin and Mucous Membrane Integrity of the Head and Neck
    c. Biologically Sound and Functional Dentition
    d. Conceptualization and Problem Solving

18 Assessment of Dental Deposits and Stain

COMPETENCIES

1. Compare and contrast the different types of oral deposits and stains.
2. Apply appropriate techniques for the assessment of dental deposits.
3. Discuss with patients the impact of dental deposits on oral health.
4. Utilize oral hygiene indices for patient assessment and education.
5. Explain the significance of record keeping and documentation as it relates to the assessment of dental deposits and stain.

SHORT ANSWER QUESTIONS

1. List the four most common gingivitis-causing bacteria.

_____

_____

_____

_____

2. List the four most common advanced periodontal disease-causing bacteria.

_____

_____

_____

_____

3. List the four most common bacteria associated with periodontal health.

_____

_____

_____

_____

4. List the stages of oral biofilm formation.

_____

_____

_____

_____

5. Describe how the patient's ability to manage oral self-care is assessed.

_____

_____

_____

6. List organic and inorganic components of calculus.

_____

_____

_____

_____

_____

_____

_____

_____

FILL IN THE BLANK STATEMENTS

Select the best term from the following list and complete the following statements.

    a. Calculus
    b. Food debris
    c. Biofilm
    d. Acquired pellicle
    e. Materia alba

1. _____ Loose mass of bacteria and cellular debris

2. _____ Organic acellular layer

3. _____ Dietary remnants/loose particles

4. _____ Mineralized matrix of bacterial colonies

5. _____ Gel-like complex matrix of bacterial colonies

Select the best term from the chapter and complete the following statements.

6. Using _____, calculus can be observed as a dark, opaque, shadowlike area against the translucent enamel.

7. A _____ is a data collection instrument that allows the clinician to convert specific clinical observations into numeric values.

8. The _____ is an index that can be used to assess the degree of oral biofilm and calculus.

Complete each question by circling the best answer.

1. All of the following are soft and hard deposit assessment descriptors EXCEPT:
   a. Amount
   b. Color
   c. Location
   d. Extent

2. The MOST common sites for calculus deposits are:
   a. Mandibular lingual molars and maxillary facial anteriors
   b. Mandibular facial molars and maxillary lingual anteriors
   c. Maxillary lingual molars and mandibular facial anteriors
   d. Maxillary facial molars and mandibular lingual anteriors

3. The ingredient in disclosing solutions that stains oral biofilm red is:
   a. Erythrosine
   b. Red dye #2
   c. Vegetable protein
   d. Natural beet juice

4. Undisturbed oral biofilm causes initial signs of gingival inflammation by:
   a. 1-3 hours
   b. 4-14 hours
   c. 1-3 days
   d. 4-14 days

5. All of the following stains may be removed by scaling and polishing EXCEPT:
   a. Stannous Fluoride
   b. Chromogenic
   c. Tetracycline
   d. Chlorhexidine gluconate

6. Your patient is a heavy tea drinker and is scheduled for his routine 6-month recare appointment. He has heavy brown stain and is concerned it may cause him to lose his teeth. His overall oral health is good with pocket depths of 2-3 mm and no loss of attachment. You explain in your oral hygiene instruction that heavy tea stain:
   a. may lead to dental decay
   b. may lead to periodontal disease
   c. is primarily an esthetic concern
   d. can cause increased calculus formation

7. Extrinsic stains can be removed by:
   a. Scaling and polishing with a mild abrasive
   b. Polishing with excessive force
   c. Using a mouthrinse containing chlorhexidine gluconate
   d. Using periodontal files

8. An amorphous film that forms over tooth surfaces and restorations and contains no bacteria is:
   a. Dental biofilm
   b. Materia alba
   c. Acquired pellicle
   d. Calculus

9. Hard deposits, soft deposits, and stain should be documented during the implementation phase of the dental hygiene care plan. When assessing soft deposits, an individualized homecare plan should include flossing.
   a. Both statements are true.
   b. Both statements are false.
   c. The first statement is true, the second statement is false.
   d. The first statement is false, the second statement is true.

10. Your patient is concerned that moderate brown stain from daily coffee consumption on anterior facial and lingual surfaces will cause decay. She is also interested in whitening her teeth. What Human Needs deficit does this address?
    a. Protection from Health Risks
    b. Wholesome Facial Image
    c. Skin and Mucous Membrane Integrity of the Head and Neck
    d. Responsibility for Oral Health

11. Which of the following stain types can be removed using ultrasonic scaling and selective polishing?
    a. Hypocalcification
    b. Fluorosis
    c. Chromogenic
    d. Tetracycline

12. Which bacteria is associated with advancing periodontal disease?
    a. Facultative
    b. Anaerobic
    c. Fusiform
    d. Aerobic

CASE STUDY

Your patient, a 35-year-old male teacher, presents to your office for routine dental hygiene therapy. It has been 3 years since his last appointment with you. He states that he has developed diabetes. Oral exam reveals heavy biofilm, BOP, and moderate calculus generalized.

1. What other dental deposits will you assess for?
2. What education plan do you have for this patient?
3. What index would be appropriate?
4. What type of bacteria is most likely present subgingivally? Supragingivally? Why?

_____

_____

_____

_____

_____

_____

_____

_____

_____

_____

_____

_____

_____

_____

_____

_____

Performance Objective

The student will demonstrate acceptable knowledge and skill evaluating patient oral deposit assessment for **18.1 Oral Deposit Assessment**.

Evaluation and Grading Criteria

Instructor will assign grades for each performance criteria.

<u>3</u> Student competently met stated criteria

<u>2</u> Student required minimal assistance to meet criteria

<u>1</u> Student showed uncertainty when attempting criteria

<u>0</u> Student was not prepared and needs to repeat criteria

<u>N/A</u> Student was not evaluated

Performance Standards

Instructor shall identify steps that are critical with an asterisk (*)

Performance Criteria	*	Self	Peer	Instructor	Comments
1. Used personal protective equipment appropriately					
2. Correct patient positioning					
3. Gathered appropriate armamentarium a. Mouth mirror b. Periodontal explorer c. Disclosing solution d. 2 × 2 gauze					
4. Appropriate use of compressed air					
5. Appropriate use of intraoral light source					
6. Patient hand mirror					
7. Oral hygiene assessment form					
8. Selection of appropriate dental index					
9. Documentation					
10. Prevention of Disease Transmission	*				
ADDITIONAL COMMENTS					

19 Dental Caries Management by Risk Assessment

COMPETENCIES

1. Explain the team approach and primary purpose in integrating caries management by risk assessment (**CAMBRA®**) into an oral health care practice.
2. Describe the caries process and relate each of the following to the dental caries process:
   (a) Process of demineralization and remineralization that occurs in the oral environment;
   (b) Saliva's beneficial actions; and
   (c) Dental caries balance.
3. Assess risk of dental caries for patients 6 years of age through adult, including the following:
   (a) Caries disease indicators;
   (b) Caries risk factors;
   (c) Caries protective factors; and
   (d) Use the caries risk assessment form and test salivary flow rate.
4. Assess level of dental caries in children from birth to 5 years of age, including the caries risk factors and the caries protective factors. Also, explain the parent/caregiver recommendations for caries prevention.
5. Use clinical guidelines for dental caries management.
6. Relate the risk level of dental caries to the indications for the several types of fluoride therapies.
7. Relate dental caries risk level to indications for evidence-based nonfluoride caries-preventive agents.
8. Discuss legal, ethical, and safety issues related to caries management, as well as future possibilities for caries management products.

SHORT ANSWER QUESTIONS

1. List benefits of saliva.

_____

_____

_____

_____

_____

_____

_____

_____

_____

2. What are the four caries disease indicators for Caries Risk Assessment?

_____

_____

_____

_____

_____

3. What are the high-risk disease indicators for children age 6 and older to adult?

_____

_____

_____

_____

_____

_____

_____

_____

_____

_____

_____

4. What are the caries risk factors for children age 6 and older to adult?

_____

_____

_____

_____

_____

_____

_____

_____

_____

_____

_____

_____

_____

5. What is the criteria for extreme caries risk for children age 6 and older to adult?

_____

_____

_____

_____

_____

_____

_____

_____

6. What are factors for high caries risk for children birth to 5 years of age?

_____

_____

_____

_____

_____

_____

_____

_____

_____

_____

_____

_____

_____

_____

_____

7. List protective factors for children birth to 5 years of age.

_____

_____

_____

_____

_____

_____

8. List the caries risk factors that contribute to new caries development or progression of existing caries.

_____

_____

_____

_____

_____

_____

_____

_____

_____

_____

FILL IN THE BLANK STATEMENTS

Select the best term from the chapter and complete the following statements.

1. _____ is a term used to describe the process or method where the clinician identifies hazards and risk factors that have the potential to cause harm.

2. _____ is an evidence-based approach to preventing or treating dental caries at the earliest stages.

3. _____ is a preventable oral disease caused by a persistent acid imbalance facilitated by oral biofilm.

4. _____ is a complex, organized microbial environment that is the primary etiologic factor for the most frequently occurring oral diseases such as dental caries and periodontal diseases.

5. _____ is a dissolution of tooth surface enamel and is the earliest stage of dental caries.

6. The presence of clinically detectable, localized areas of enamel demineralization is considered a _____

_____.

7. A deposition of minerals into demineralized areas of tooth structure that repairs an initial carious lesion is _____

_____.

8. _____ is a method to predict future caries development before the clinical onset of the disease.

9. _____ an infectious disease that affects children from birth to 2 years of age and rapidly destroys newly erupted teeth.

10. _____ is the persistence of effect of a topically applied drug, determined by the degree of physical and chemical bonding to the surface and the resistance to removal or inactivation.

11. Demineralization of tooth structure occurs at or below a pH of _____.

MULTIPLE CHOICE QUESTIONS

Complete each question by circling the best answer.

1. Topical fluoride should be placed following complete scaling and prophylaxis. The reduction of oral biofilm thickness facilitates the diffusion of fluoride to the enamel surface.
   a. Both statements are true.
   b. Both statements are false.
   c. The first statement is true and the second statement is false.
   d. The first statement is false and the second statement is true.

2. Xylitol is not fermented by cariogenic bacteria. Xylitol is a sugar alcohol that moderately affects glycemic index.
   a. Both statements are true.
   b. Both statements are false.
   c. The first statement is true and the second statement is false.
   d. The first statement is false and the second statement is true.

3. A caries lesion that develops at the margin of an existing restoration is:
   a. Primary
   b. Secondary
   c. Tertiary
   d. Residual

4. In the early stages of dental caries formation, the process can be arrested. Once the caries process begins, it cannot be reversed.
   a. Both statements are truc.
   b. Both statements are false.
   c. The first statement is true and the second statement is false.
   d. The first statement is false and the second statement is true.

5. Research shows that levels of fluoride can be observed up to 6 months after application. The introduction of fluoride has contributed to the decline in caries rates without major changes in sugar consumption.
   a. Both statements are true.
   b. Both statements are false.
   c. The first statement is true and the second statement is false.
   d. The first statement is false and the second statement is true.

6. Caries can be modified by protective factors. Current research supports providing topical fluoride to all patients with moderate and high risk for caries.
   a. Both statements are true.
   b. Both statements are false.
   c. The first statement is true and the second statement is false.
   d. The first statement is false and the second statement is true.

7. Your patient presents with no current active carious lesions, and no restorations have been placed due to caries in the last 5 years. Your patient states she has frequent dry mouth, verified with a saliva test. What risk for caries is your patient using the Caries Risk Assessment as a guide?
   a. Low
   b. Moderate
   c. High
   d. Severe

8. Your patient presents for their recare visit, and he is diagnosed with two new carious lesions since his last 6-month visit. He had one carious lesion restored 6 months ago. His caries risk is:
   a. Low
   b. Moderate
   c. High
   d. Extreme

9. Caries Risk Assessment determines the probability of a new caries incident. Caries Risk Assessment determines the probability that there will be a change in activity or size of carious lesions.
   a. Both statements are true.
   b. Both statements are false.
   c. The first statement is true and the second statement is false.
   d. The first statement is false and the second statement is true.

10. Demineralization is the loss of calcium and enamel in tooth structure. Enamel can repair itself by using calcium ions incorporate into the remineralizing tooth structure.
    a. Both statements are true.
    b. Both statements are false.
    c. The first statement is true and the second statement is false.
    d. The first statement is false and the second statement is true.

11. Normal pH of the oral cavity is approximately 7 or neutral. Acids produced by bacteria in response to sugar cause normal pH to drop below 5.5.
    a. Both statements are true.
    b. Both statements are false.
    c. The first statement is true and the second statement is false.
    d. The first statement is false and the second statement is true.

12. Your 20-year-old patient has several areas of caries. After reviewing her dietary analysis, you notice she has several potentially carious causes. Which of the following is most likely responsible for her high caries rate?
    a. Lives in an area with no municipal fluoride water supply
    b. She drinks several cans of soda a day, sipping throughout the day
    c. She drinks 1 cup of coffee with 1 teaspoon of sugar and 2 tablespoons of milk in the morning
    d. She brushes with a "natural" toothpaste that contains no fluoride

13. How long does it take for pH level to return to normal after ingesting fermentable carbohydrates?
    a. 10-20 minutes
    b. 30-60 minutes
    c. 1-3 days
    d. 7-14 days

CASE STUDY #1

Three-year-old Thomas has no visible signs of caries. He has no significant family history of caries. His father reports that Thomas has a sippy cup of orange juice in the morning and a cup of apple juice in the afternoon. His snacks are usually apple slices, string cheese, and crackers. Thomas has no siblings. They reside in an area with no fluoridated water.

What is Thomas's caries risk?
What are the recommendations for caries prevention?
What are some education topics to cover during OHI?

_____

_____

_____

_____

_____

_____

_____

_____

_____

_____

_____

_____

_____

CASE STUDY #2

Four-year-old Samantha has Down Syndrome and needs assistance with daily oral care. She has no apparent caries and has visible biofilm on anterior teeth. Samantha's caregiver states it is a challenge keeping up with Samantha's home care.

What is Samantha's caries risk?
What is Thomas's caries risk?
What are some recommendations for caries prevention?
What are some education topics to cover during OHI?

_____

_____

_____

_____

_____

_____

_____

_____

_____

_____

_____

_____

CASE STUDY #3

Seven-year-old Buddy received stainless steel crowns on two primary teeth when he was 5 years old. He has several white-spot lesions. His 10-year-old sister and his father have had multiple restorations. The family sporadically reports for routine oral care. Moderate biofilm is present on Buddy's teeth.

What is Buddy's caries risk?
What are some recommendations for caries prevention?
What are some education topics to cover during OHI?

_____

_____

_____

_____

_____

_____

_____

_____

_____

_____

CASE STUDY #4

Ten-year-old Yulia recently moved to the US from Ukraine. She has never had an oral exam or been to the dentist. She has several white spot lesions. She has moderate visible biofilm. Fluoride exposure in undetermined. Family history is undeterminable, since no one has ever seen a dentist.

What is Yulia's caries risk?
What are some recommendations for caries prevention?
What are some education topics to cover during OHI?

_____

_____

_____

_____

_____

_____

_____

_____

_____

_____

Performance Objective

By following a routine procedure that meets the stated protocols, the student will demonstrate the appropriate technique for **Procedure 19-1 Use of the Caries Risk Assessment Form**

Evaluation and Grading Criteria

Instructor will assign grades for each performance criteria.

<u>3</u> Student competently met stated criteria

<u>2</u> Student required minimal assistance to meet criteria

<u>1</u> Student showed uncertainty when attempting criteria

<u>0</u> Student was not prepared and needs to repeat criteria

<u>N/A</u> Student was not evaluated

Performance Standards

Instructor shall identify steps that are critical with an asterisk (*)

Performance Criteria	*	Self	Peer	Instructor	Comments
1. Based on data obtained from the health histories and clinical examination, circle the *Yes* categories in the three columns on the Caries Risk Assessment form					
2. Make notations regarding the number of carious lesions present, the oral hygiene status, the brand of fluorides used, the type of snacks eaten, and the names of medications or drugs causing dry mouth.					
3. If the answer is *Yes* to any one of the four disease indicators in the first column, then take a bacterial culture using the Caries Risk Test (see Procedure 18-2) (Ivoclar Vivadent, Amherst, New York) or an equivalent test.					
4. Make an overall judgment as to whether the patient is at low, moderate, high, or extreme risk depending on the balance between the disease indicators or risk factors and the protective factors using the caries balance concept. *Patients who have a current caries lesion or had one in the recent past are at high risk for future caries. Patients who are at high risk and have severe salivary gland hypofunction or special needs are at extreme risk and require very intensive therapy. If the patient is not at high or low risk, then he or she by default is at moderate risk.					
ADDITIONAL COMMENTS					

Performance Objective

By following a routine procedure that meets the stated protocols, the student will demonstrate the appropriate technique for **Procedure 19-2 Testing Salivary Flow Rate and Level of Caries Bacterial Challenge**

Evaluation and Grading Criteria

Instructor will assign grades for each performance criteria.

> 3 Student competently met stated criteria
>
> 2 Student required minimal assistance to meet criteria
>
> 1 Student showed uncertainty when attempting criteria
>
> 0 Student was not prepared and needs to repeat criteria

N/A Student was not evaluated

Performance Standards

Instructor shall identify steps that are critical with an asterisk (*)

Performance Criteria	*	Self	Peer	Instructor	Comments
5. Equipment ■ Paraffin pellets ■ Measuring cup ■ Commercially available caries bacterial test kit, such as the Caries Risk Test ■ Incubator ■ Personal protective barriers					
Determine salivary flow rate: 6. Have the patient chew a paraffin pellet for 3 to 5 minutes (timed) and spit all saliva generated into a measuring cup.					
7. At the end of the 3 to 5 minutes, measure the amount of saliva in milliliters (mL) and divide that amount by time to determine the mL/min of stimulated salivary flow.					
8. A flow rate of 1 mL/min or higher is considered normal; a level of 0.7 mL/min is low; and anything at 0.5 mL/min or less is dry, indicating severe salivary gland hypofunction.					
9. Investigate the reason for the flow rate if it is 0.7 mL/min or less (medication, radiation, systemic condition).					
Initiate bacterial testing: 10. The kit comes with a two-sided selective media stick that assesses mutans streptococci (MS) on the blue side and lactobacilli (LB) on the green side.					
11. Remove the selective media stick from the culture tube. Peel off the plastic cover sheet from each side of the stick.					

Continued

Performance Criteria	*	Self	Peer	Instructor	Comments
12. Pour (do not streak) the collected saliva over the media on each side until it is entirely wet.					
13. Place one of the sodium bicarbonate tablets included in the kit in the bottom of the tube.					
14. Replace the media stick in the culture tube, screw the lid on, and label the tube with the patient's name, registration number, and date.					
15. Prevention of Disease Transmission	*				
ADDITIONAL COMMENTS					

20 Periodontal Assessment and Charting

COMPETENCIES

1. Relate periodontal assessment and its significance to the dental hygiene process of care.
2. Discuss the four physical units of a healthy periodontium, as well as the clinical signs and histologic characteristics of a healthy and diseased periodontium.
3. Discuss periodontal diseases, including characteristics/signs, types, and causes. Also, classify periodontal diseases using the classification systems of the American Academy of Periodontology (AAP) and the European Federation of Periodontology (EFP).
4. Perform thorough and accurate periodontal assessment of the periodontium and implants.
5. Discuss risk factors for periodontal diseases and their relationship stages and grades of periodontitis and dental hygiene care planning.
6. Explain proper documentation and record keeping for periodontal assessment and treatment.

SHORT ANSWER QUESTIONS

1. List the four aspects of a healthy periodontium.

_____

_____

_____

_____

2. List the four anatomical aspects of the gingiva.

_____

_____

_____

_____

3. Briefly describe Clinical Attachment Loss (CAL).

_____

_____

_____

_____

4. What are the two distinct causes of periodontal destruction?

_____

_____

_____

_____

111

5. What are the four clinical characteristic signs of gingival or periodontal inflammation?

_____

_____

_____

_____

_____

FILL IN THE BLANK STATEMENTS

Select the best term from the chapter and complete the following statements.

1. _____ is secreted from the connective tissue within the sulcus.

2. The _____ is fibrous connective tissue within the gingival sulcus.

3. _____ is a reversible bacterial infection confined to gingiva only with no migration of junctional epithelium.

4. A _____ occurs when the junctional epithelium migrates beyond the cementoenamel junction but stays above the crest of the alveolar bone. This is also known as _____.

5. An _____ occurs when the junctional epithelium migrates below the crest of the alveolar bone. This is also known as _____.

MULTIPLE CHOICE QUESTIONS

Complete each question by circling the best answer.

1. Gingival diseases may be modified by all of the following EXCEPT:
   a. Medication
   b. Systemic factors
   c. Viral origin
   d. Environmental

2. When documenting clinical gingival assessment, all of the following terms are used to describe gingival changes EXCEPT:
   a. Quantity
   b. Distribution
   c. Severity
   d. Location

3. Which of the following would be a modifiable risk factor for periodontal disease?
   a. Diabetes
   b. Tobacco
   c. HIV
   d. Stress

4. What classification of mobility describes a tooth that can be moved in any direction but not depressible?
   a. 1
   b. 2
   c. 3
   d. 4

5. What furcation classification allows the clinician to use a Nabor's probe to enter a furcation space from the facial aspect of a tooth but not penetrate through to the lingual aspect?
   a. I
   b. II
   c. III
   d. IV

6. A reduction of height of the marginal gingiva to a location apical to the CEJ is:
   a. Fremitus
   b. Furcation
   c. Inadequate attached gingiva (IAG)
   d. Recession

7. Measuring from the free gingival margin to the mucogingival junction renders which periodontal finding?
   a. Width of attachment
   b. Recession
   c. Furcation
   d. Fremitus

8. All of the following are local contributing factors to periodontal disease EXCEPT:
   a. Tongue piercing
   b. Restoration with open contact
   c. Tooth malposition
   d. Diabetes

9. IAG includes all of the following statements EXCEPT:
   a. The presence of less than 1 mm of keratinized attached gingiva
   b. Is measured on the facial aspects of mandibular teeth
   c. Is measured on the palatal side of maxillary teeth
   d. Recession may be involved

10. A patient reports with severe periodontal disease, type I diabetes and heart disease. Discussing the correlation of oral health and overall health addresses what Human Needs Model deficit?
   a. Protection from Health Risks
   b. Biologically Sound and Functional Dentition
   c. Conceptualization and Problem Solving
   d. Responsibility for Oral Health

11. If a pocket depth measures 6 mm and recession measures 2 mm, what is the CAL?
   a. 2 mm
   b. 4 mm
   c. 6 mm
   d. 8 mm

12. Which of the following is a nonmodifiable risk factor for periodontal disease?
   a. Gender
   b. Tobacco use
   c. Obesity
   d. Stress

CASE STUDY

A 30-year-old new patient reports for her initial exam. Findings include:

- Health History reveals BP 150/90
  - No medical care or routine oral care in over 10 years
  - Patient reports a family history of diabetes, cardiovascular disease, and periodontal disease
  - Patient smokes 1 pack of cigarettes a day
  - Patient may be pregnant
  - No current meds
- Oral exam/dental exam reveals
  - generalized moderate biofilm supra and sub
  - generalized calculus supra and sub
  - 6-7 mm pocket depths post, 4-6 mm pocket depths
  - Generalized BOP and moderate-severe inflammation
  - #19 needs endodontic treatment
  - #30 has decay on the occlusal
  - patient reports pain with #31–has severe decay and needs extraction

1. What radiographs, if any, would you expose?
2. What is her dental hygiene diagnosis?
3. What education plan would you provide?
4. What other diagnostic tests would you conduct, if any?

_____

_____

_____

_____

_____

_____

_____

_____

_____

_____

_____

_____

_____

_____

21 Oral-Systemic Health Connection

COMPETENCIES

1. Explain why the oral-systemic health connection is important in providing evidence-based care, and discuss how cardiovascular disease, diabetes, and pregnancy can affect oral health.
2. Incorporate periodontal-systemic evidence into treatment and practice and educate patients about areas of association between periodontal disease and systemic disease, as well as how these associations influence the patient's risk of developing periodontal disease and/or systemic disease. Also, determine the need for referrals to primary care providers for dental patients with systemic disease.

SHORT ANSWER QUESTIONS

1. List the three criteria needed to determine a causal relationship.

_____

_____

_____

_____

2. Which classification of pneumonia involves a patient acquiring pneumonia within 48 hours of admission into a hospital stay?

_____

_____

3. List the diseases that have a moderate bidirectional association with periodontal disease.

_____

_____

_____

_____

4. What is the common association between periodontal disease and systemic diseases?

_____

_____

5. List and briefly describe the types of respiratory diseases.

_____

_____

_____

_____

_____

6. Identify and briefly describe the biological plausibility theories between adverse pregnancy outcomes and periodontitis.

_____

_____

_____

_____

_____

FILL IN THE BLANK STATEMENTS

Select the best term from the chapter and complete the following statements.

1. Association of normal living processes is _____.

2. _____ reflects a patient's blood glucose control over the past several months.

3. _____ is a systemic marker for inflammation.

4. Preterm birth is considered at _____ weeks before expected delivery.

5. _____ is a lung infection resulting from inhaling saliva.

Complete each question by circling the best answer.

1. The criteria to determine a causal relationship between two diseases is also known as:
   a. Oral/Systemic Health Status
   b. Angles Assessment
   c. Overall Health Assessment
   d. Bradford Hill Research

2. All of the following may have a bidirectional association with the progression of periodontal disease EXCEPT:
   a. Diabetes
   b. Asthma
   c. Low birth weight
   d. Cardiovascular disease

3. It is safe to take oral radiographs and provide therapeutic dental procedures during pregnancy. Oral radiographs and therapeutic dental procedures can only be provided during the third trimester.
   a. Both statements are true.
   b. Both statements are false.
   c. The first statement is true, the second statement is false.
   d. The first statement is false, the second statement is true.

4. Research demonstrates a weak association between periodontal disease and certain systemic diseases. These weak associations negates a causal relationship.
   a. Both statements are true.
   b. Both statements are false.
   c. The first statement is true, the second statement is false.
   d. The first statement is false, the second statement is true.

5. All of the following are pneumonia classifications EXCEPT:
   a. CAP
   b. HAP
   c. VAP
   d. PAP

6. The inability of the body to utilize produced insulin is:
   a. Type I diabetes
   b. Type II diabetes
   c. HbA1c
   d. Pancreatic parafunction

7. Patients with diabetes have difficulty controlling gingival inflammation. Patients with gingival inflammation have difficulty controlling blood glucose levels.
   a. Both statements are true.
   b. Both statements are false.
   c. The first statement is true, the second statement is false.
   d. The first statement is false, the second statement is true.

8. What is the BEST Human Needs Conceptual Model deficit that addresses a patient with uncontrolled diabetes and severe periodontal disease?
   a. Wholesome Facial Image
   b. Skin and Mucous Membrane Integrity of the Head and Neck
   c. Biologically Sound and Functional Dentition
   d. Conceptualization and Problem Solving

9. When dental hygienists seek evidence-based research supporting an association between periodontal disease and systemic diseases, which are the BEST types of studies to look for?
   a. Longitudinal intervention human studies
   b. Case studies
   c. Observational studies
   d. Correlational studies

10. All of the following are risk factors for diabetes and CVD EXCEPT:
    a. Genetic predisposition
    b. Obesity
    c. Poor oral hygiene
    d. Limited physical activity

11. Strong evidence supports an association between which types of respiratory diseases?
    a. VAP and HAP
    b. CAP and VAP
    c. AP only
    d. CAP only

12. Which of the following conditions demonstrates limited research supporting a connection to periodontitis?
    a. HAP
    b. CVD
    c. Diabetes
    d. COPD

CASE STUDY

Your 60-year-old male patient, Mr. H, presents to your office as a referral from his cardiologist. Mr. H had a heart attack 2 months ago. He smokes 1 pack of cigarettes a day and is interested in quitting. His last dental exam was over 10 years ago. Comprehensive oral exam and dental hygiene diagnosis reveal generalized severe chronic periodontal disease. Pocket depths are 5-7 mm with bleeding. Heavy subgingival calculus and moderate biofilm are present generalized. Tooth numbers 23-26 have class II mobility. Class II furcations are present on all molars. He reports brushing once a day and occasionally uses a toothpick interproximally.

Develop a detailed treatment plan for Mr. H.

- What educational plan do you propose?
- What are his short-term goals?
- What are his long-term goals?
- How will the treatment you provide impact his overall health?

Dental Hygiene Diagnosis

COMPETENCIES

1. Compare and contrast a dental hygiene and a dental diagnosis using nursing and medicine as a parallel.
2. Discuss the dental hygiene diagnostic process in action and apply the Human Needs and Oral Health-Related Quality of Life models for decision making in the development of a dental hygiene diagnosis.
3. Implement the dental hygiene diagnostic process by identifying interventions that support various dental hygiene diagnoses, write dental hygiene diagnoses, and educate and motivate clients to work toward positive behavior changes.
4. Gather complete data during patient assessment to support recognizable patterns in formulating diagnoses – demonstrating validation and support for the process in providing individualized dental hygiene care.
5. Discuss the outcomes and benefits of dental hygiene diagnoses.

SHORT ANSWER QUESTIONS

1. How is the dental hygiene diagnosis different from the dental diagnosis?

_____

_____

_____

_____

2. List various work settings for the dental hygienist.

_____

_____

_____

_____

_____

_____

3. What method do practitioners use to systematically follow their care of patients?

_____

_____

_____

_____

4. Which diagnostic decision-making model uses deficits in a patient's oral health/overall health along with patient goals and dental hygiene interventions?

_____

_____

_____

_____

5. To validate a dental hygiene diagnosis, what must the dental hygienist compare?

_____

_____

_____

_____

6. List the five aspects of dental hygiene diagnosis according to ADHA *Standards for Clinical Dental Hygiene Practice* Standard 2.

_____

_____

_____

_____

_____

_____

_____

_____

FILL IN THE BLANK STATEMENTS

Select the best term from the chapter and complete the following statements.

1. Conscious use of current best research in deciding patient care is _____.

2. _____ is diagnosed based on biological, social, and psychological data.

3. _____ is the state of complete physical, mental, and social well-being.

4. _____ is a multidimensional construct that reflects people's comfort when eating, sleeping, and engaging in social interaction; their self-esteem; and their satisfaction with respect to their oral health.

5. _____ is a person-centered psychotherapeutic approach that moves a patient away from a state of indecision or uncertainty and toward finding motivation to making positive decisions and accomplishing established goals.

6. _____ is the ability of the dental hygienist to initiate treatment based on the assessment of a patient's needs without the specific authorization of a dentist.

Complete each question by circling the best answer.

1. A diagnosis that targets a disease or condition is:
   a. Medical
   b. Dental
   c. Nursing
   d. Dental hygiene

2. A diagnosis that addresses a patient's response to illness and family impact is:
   a. Medical
   b. Dental
   c. Nursing
   d. Dental hygiene

3. A diagnosis that targets oral disease is:
   a. Medical
   b. Dental
   c. Nursing
   d. Dental hygiene

4. A diagnosis that seeks to prevent oral disease, minimizes risk of oral disease, and promotes wellness is:
   a. Medical
   b. Dental
   c. Nursing
   d. Dental hygiene

5. Medicine and dentistry function within the classic biomedical, disease-oriented approach to care. Nursing and dental hygiene use a holistic approach to care that encourages patient-clinician collaboration.
   a. Both statements are true.
   b. Both statements are false.
   c. The first statement is true, the second statement is false.
   d. The first statement is false, the second statement is true.

6. According to the ADHA, a dental hygiene diagnosis includes all of the following EXCEPT:
   a. Requires evidence-based critical analysis and interpretation
   b. Is the framework for the dental treatment plan
   c. Identifies health behaviors, attitudes, and oral health care needs of patients
   d. Must be carried out by a licensed provider

7. The dental hygiene process of care includes all of the following EXCEPT:
   a. Assess
   b. Implement
   c. Evaluate
   d. Diagnose

8. The ability of a dental hygienist to begin patient care without the authorization of a dentist and treat without a dentist present is:
   a. Direct access
   b. Indirect access
   c. Remote access
   d. Full access

9. Dental hygiene diagnosis was developed because:
   a. Dental diagnosis is incomplete
   b. All professions have their own separate diagnoses
   c. Dental hygienists may work independently
   d. Dental hygiene schools require dental hygiene diagnosis in the curriculum

10. Which of the following is NOT included in the dental hygiene diagnosis?
    a. Radiographs
    b. Medical history
    c. Clinical evaluation
    d. Social determinants

11. Oral health–related quality-of-life model includes traditional collection of data as well as biological/psychological and social determinants of health. Oral health–related quality-of-life model is included in the development of the dental hygiene diagnosis.
    a. Both statements are true.
    b. Both statements are false.
    c. The first statement is true, the second statement is false.
    d. The first statement is false, the second statement is true.

12. A patient presents with severe fluorosis and is interested in veneers. What Human Needs Conceptual model deficit does this address?
    a. Freedom from Fear and Stress
    b. Wholesome Facial Image
    c. Biologically Sound and Functional Dentition
    d. Responsibility for Oral Health

13. A patient presents with severe gingivitis. What Human Needs Conceptual model deficit does this address?
    a. Protection from Health Risks
    b. Freedom from Pain
    c. Skin and Mucous Membrane Integrity of the Head and Neck
    d. Responsibility for Oral Health

Age	32	SCENARIO
Gender	female	**EOE/IOE:**
Height	5'9"	Coated tongue
Weight	210 lb	Moderate biofilm generalized
B/P	170/105 mm Hg	Moderate calculus generalized
Chief Complaint	Pain in upper left quadrant, cold and hot sensitivity, halitosis	Moderate extrinsic brown stain generalized
Medical History	Family history of cardiovascular disease Patient has not seen her family physician in over a year	**Periodontal Findings:** Generalized bleeding on probing Probe readings 5-6 posterior, 3-4 anterior Type III periodontitis Chronic gingival inflammation
Current Medications	Hydrochlorothiazide 20 mg daily	**Radiographic Findings:** Endodontic lesion #14
Social History	Drinks 2-3 glasses of beer daily

Patient works as a waitress in a local restaurant. She has 2 children and a very busy life.

She admits to not always eating healthy and tends to snack on sweets. She drinks 3 glasses of sweet tea daily and 2 cups of coffee with cream and sugar. She also admits to sporadically taking prescribed meds | **Dental Findings:** Caries present in #14 MOD, #18 O

Last dental exam 4 years ago. She rates her oral health as poor. She has had bad experiences with dental treatment in the past and is fearful about today's appointment. She is not satisfied with the dark appearance of her teeth.

She reports brushing once a day and does not use floss or any device for interdental biofilm removal. |

Using the data from this patient, develop a Human Needs Conceptual model for treatment.

Dental Hygiene Diagnosis (unmet human need)	Etiology (due to…)	Signs and Symptoms (evidenced by…)	Patient Goals (expected outcomes)
Protection from Health Risks			
Freedom from Fear and Stress			
Freedom from Pain			
Wholesome Facial Image			
Skin and Mucous Membrane Integrity of the Head and Neck			
Biologically Sound and Functional Dentition			
Conceptualization and Problem Solving			
Responsibility for Oral Health			

23 Dental Hygiene Care Plan, Evaluation, and Documentation

COMPETENCIES

1. Define the planning step of the process of care and differentiate between the dental treatment plan and the dental hygiene care plan. Also, discuss the concept of interprofessional collaboration.
2. Discuss the sequence of events in dental hygiene care plan development and, given a case scenario, formulate and evaluate a dental hygiene care plan including:
   - Link the care plan to one or more dental hygiene diagnoses.
   - Write care plan goals.
   - Select professional and self-care intervention strategies.
   - Develop an appointment schedule.
   - Determine attainment of care plan outcomes and write a supportive evaluation statement.
3. Discuss the care plan presentation, maximizing patient involvement and the patient's potential informed consent and informed refusal as related to dental hygiene care planning.
4. Define the goal of evaluation in the process of care and explain the importance of measuring care plan outcomes including:
   - Discuss how evaluation is integrated into the dental hygiene process of care.
   - Discuss evaluation strategies for monitoring and measuring achievement of care plan outcomes.
5. Discuss documentation in the dental record and its significance to the process of care.

SHORT ANSWER QUESTIONS

1. Describe the ADHA Standard 3: Planning. Include its purpose.

_____

_____

_____

_____

_____

2. Describe the difference between and dental treatment plan and a dental hygiene care plan.

_____

_____

_____

_____

_____

3. Briefly explain the Human Needs Conceptual Model (HN).

_____

_____

_____

_____

4. Briefly explain the Oral Heath Related Quality of Life Model (OHRQL).

_____

_____

_____

_____

5. Explain the goal of ADHA Standard 5: Evaluation.

_____

_____

_____

_____

6. List the four types of patient goal categories.

_____

_____

_____

_____

7. List the steps in Evaluation of Care.

_____

_____

_____

_____

_____

_____

8. List possible patient-centered barriers to personal health and wellness.

_____

_____

_____

_____

_____

_____

_____

_____

_____

_____

FILL IN THE BLANK STATEMENTS

Select the best term from the chapter and complete the following statements.

1. _____ is a process of providing a patient with the information needed to the make a decision about treatment that includes a comprehensive discussion with the health care provider regarding the proposed care plan and risks of not receiving care.

2. _____ is when a patient has refused a recommended treatment based upon an understanding of the facts and implications of not following the treatment.

3. _____ is the process of continual review and reinforcement of patient progress toward goals.

4. The complete and accurate recording of all collected data, care planned and provided, patient consent for treatment, treatment outcomes, continued care recommendations, and other interactions and information relevant to patient care

   is _____.

5. _____ is a continuous process of reviewing and interpreting the outcome of implemented care.

MULTIPLE CHOICE QUESTIONS

Complete each question by circling the best answer.

1. A goal category that targets a patient's mastery of dental floss is:
   a. Cognitive
   b. Psychomotor
   c. Affective
   d. Oral health status

2. A goal category that targets the patient's appreciation of the importance of supplemental fluoride to assist in caries reduction is:
   a. Cognitive
   b. Psychomotor
   c. Affective
   d. Oral health status

3. A goal category that targets the patient's decrease in bleeding upon probing after nonsurgical periodontal therapy is:
   a. Cognitive
   b. Psychomotor
   c. Affective
   d. Oral health status

4. All of the following support establishing the parameters for evaluation in the dental hygiene process of care EXCEPT:
   a. Assess
   b. Diagnose
   c. Plan
   d. Implement

5. The dental hygiene care plan includes dental hygiene diagnoses, goals, and interventions independent of the dental treatment plan. The dental treatment plan includes the dental diagnosis, all essential phases of therapy to be carried out by the dentist, dental hygienist, and patient, as well as the prognosis.
   a. Both statements are true.
   b. Both statements are false.
   c. The first statement is true, the second statement is false.
   d. The first statement is false, the second statement is true.

6. Which component of the dental hygiene care plan guides the development of the goal statement?
   a. Dental hygiene diagnosis
   b. Care plan goals
   c. Oral self-care strategies
   d. Intervention strategies

7. All of the following are strategies to assist the patient toward meeting goals EXCEPT:
   a. Care plan goals
   b. Oral self-care strategies
   c. Intervention strategies
   d. Appointment plan

8. An acceptable care plan goal will have a subject, verb, specific criteria that is measurable, and a time parameter for the goal to be met. Which of the following best describes the criteria?
   a. Action desired of the patient to achieve a desired outcome
   b. Desired observable behavior of outcome
   c. Who is responsible for the outcome
   d. When the desired patient outcome will be achieved

9. According to the Human Needs Conceptual Theory, which component of a dental hygiene diagnosis for an *unmet human need* defines the contributors to the unmet human need?
   a. Unmet need statement
   b. Etiology
   c. Signs/symptoms or evidence of the unmet need
   d. Problem statement

10. The Oral Health–Related Quality of Life model proposes setting patient-centered goals and clinical goals. Clinical goals represent the patient's desired oral health outcomes. Patient-centered goals measure cognitive, psychomotor, and affective goals.
    a. Both statements are true.
    b. Both statements are false.
    c. The first statement is true, the second statement is false.
    d. The first statement is false, the second statement is true.

11. All of the following are considered when scheduling appointments for planned dental hygiene interventions EXCEPT:
    a. Amount of time needed
    b. Number of visits
    c. Supplies needed
    d. What intervention will be addressed

12. All of the following are included in the presentation of the dental hygiene care plan EXCEPT:
    a. Potential risks
    b. Diagnosis
    c. Prognosis
    d. Treatment options

Age	15	SCENARIO
Gender	male	
Height	5'7"	**EOE/IOE:**
Weight	130 lb	Chapped lips
B/P	110/60 mm Hg	Acne
Chief Complaint	"my gums bleed when I brush"	**Periodontal Findings:**
Medical History	Hernia surgery as an infant	Probe readings WNL Moderate biofilm generalized Moderate gingival inflammation generalized
Current Medications	None	**Radiographic Findings:** No significant findings
Social History	Plays high school soccer Active in the Boy Scouts Patents are divorced, lives with his mother, sees his father once a month	**Dental Findings:** White spot lesions max anterior cervical Occlusal caries #30 Pt admits to infrequent brushing Does not use any interdental device Reports drinking 3-4 energy drinks a day

Using the data from this patient, develop a Human Needs Conceptual model for treatment.

Dental Hygiene Diagnosis (unmet human need)	Etiology (due to…)	Signs and Symptoms (evidenced by…)	Patient Goals (expected outcomes)
Protection from Health Risks			
Freedom from Fear and Stress			
Freedom from Pain			
Wholesome Facial Image			
Skin and Mucous Membrane Integrity of the Head and Neck			
Biologically Sound and Functional Dentition			
Conceptualization and Problem Solving			
Responsibility for Oral Health			

24 Toothbrushing

COMPETENCIES

1. Describe characteristics of acceptable manual toothbrush designs.
2. Describe characteristics and modes of action of power toothbrush designs.
3. Discuss toothbrushing instruction, including differentiation among toothbrushing methods including indications, limitations, and impact on oral tissues.
4. Discuss soft- and hard-tissue lesions, including factors associated with tissue lesions, and the significance of a clean tongue and toothbrush.
5. Discuss the dental hygiene process of care and toothbrushing, including the sharing of evidence-based decision making with patients regarding selection and use of a toothbrush based on specific patient needs.

SHORT ANSWER QUESTIONS

1. List several characteristics of an effective toothbrush.

_____

_____

_____

_____

_____

_____

2. List indications for patients to use a power toothbrush.

_____

_____

_____

_____

_____

_____

_____

_____

3. List the modes of action for power toothbrushes.

_____

_____

_____

_____

_____

_____

4. The dental hygienist listens to and allows the patient's participation in decision making and to respect the patient's right to make a decision. This is an example of what ethical principle?

_____

_____

_____

5. The dental hygienist allows time for self-care instruction, repetition, reinforcement, and continual assessment of each patient's oral health practices. This is an example of what ethical principle?

_____

_____

_____

_____

6. List various modes to prevent pathogenic bacterial toothbrush contamination.

_____

_____

_____

_____

_____

FILL IN THE BLANK STATEMENTS

Select the best term from the chapter and complete the following statements.

1. Wearing away of tooth surface at the CEJ due to toothbrushing is _____.

2. Excessive occlusal force causing non-carious cervical lesions is _____.

3. _____ is an inanimate object that transmits pathogenic organisms.

4. Toothbrush replacement should be based on _____.

5. Research suggests recommended brushing time to be a minimum of _____.

1. Toothbrush filaments are typically made of:
   a. Nylon
   b. Plastic
   c. Hemp
   d. Rubber

2. Vertical bristles remove biofilm more efficiently than angled BECAUSE they reach further into interproximal spaces.
   a. Both parts of the statement are true.
   b. Both parts of the statement are false.
   c. The first part is true, the second is false.
   d. The first part is false, the second is true.

3. Research supports that using excessive force with a power toothbrush causes tissue damage. Pressure applied using a power toothbrush is more than a manual toothbrush.
   a. Both statements are true.
   b. Both statements are false.
   c. The first statement is true, the second statement is false.
   d. The first statement is false, the second statement is true.

4. Modified Bass toothbrushing includes all of the following techniques EXCEPT:
   a. Aims at the sulcus
   b. Aims at the cervical area
   c. Least effective on smooth surfaces
   d. Least effective on interproximal surfaces

5. When brushing on facial and lingual surfaces of posterior teeth, toothbrush head is parallel to the arch. When brushing on facial and lingual surfaces of anterior teeth, toothbrush head is parallel to the long axis of the tooth.
   a. Both statements are true.
   b. Both statements are false.
   c. The first statement is true, the second statement is false.
   d. The first statement is false, the second statement is true.

6. Gingival trauma from toothbrushing is caused from all of the following EXCEPT:
   a. Horizontal scrubbing
   b. Bristle firmness
   c. Excessive toothbrushing
   d. Using Stillmans technique

7. The toothbrushing technique that includes filaments at a 45-degree angle into the sulcus using gentle vibratory strokes while keeping toothbrush into the sulcus is:
   a. Modified Bass
   b. Charters
   c. Stillmans
   d. Fones

8. The toothbrushing technique that includes placing filaments partially on adjacent gingiva using short, back-and-forth vibratory strokes while moving brush head occlusally is:
   a. Bass
   b. Charters
   c. Stillmans
   d. Fones

9. All of the following are characteristics of Charters toothbrushing technique EXCEPT:
   a. Filaments are directed toward the gingival margin
   b. Filaments are placed at the gingival margin
   c. Filaments are angled 45 degrees to the long axis of the tooth
   d. Short back-and-forth vibratory strokes are used for activation

10. Fones toothbrushing technique uses a vertical motion. Fones is recommended for small children with primary teeth.
    a. Both statements are true.
    b. Both statements are false.
    c. The first statement is true, the second statement is false.
    d. The first statement is false, the second statement is true.

11. Selecting a personalized toothbrushing method for patients should include all of the following EXCEPT:
    a. Needs of the patient
    b. Patient's plaque level
    c. Preference
    d. Dexterity

12. Your patient has abfraction apparent on all maxillary molars and premolars. What Human Needs Conceptual model deficit does this reflect?
    a. Protection from Health Risks
    b. Skin and Mucous Membrane Integrity of the Head and Neck
    c. Biologically Sound and Functional Dentition
    d. Responsibility for Oral Health

13. Daily use of a dentifrice with toothbrushing provides all of the following EXCEPT:
    a. Stain prevention
    b. Clean mouth feel
    c. Fluoride application
    d. Biofilm removal

14. Oral hygiene instruction should be provided to the patient:
    a. Before periodontal charting
    b. After periodontal therapy
    c. At every dental hygiene appointment
    d. Annually

15. All of the following is true concerning power toothbrushes EXCEPT:
    a. They are effective
    b. They are safe
    c. They can be used by almost everyone
    d. They should be replaced every 6 months

16. How often should a patient brush per day?
    a. Once
    b. Twice
    c. Three times
    d. There is no set frequency

CASE STUDY: MS. BLACKSTONE

Age	24	SCENARIO
Gender	female	
Height	5'4"	**EOE/IOE:**
Weight	130 lb	Crepitus bilateral
B/P	110/70 mm Hg	
Chief Complaint	sensitivity on facial surfaces	**Periodontal Findings:** Probe readings WNL, minimal bleeding, generalized 2-3 mm recession facially
Medical History Current Medications	Achilles tendon surgery 2018 Obsessive compulsive disorder Yasmin birth control daily Prozac daily	Firm, pink tissue Festooning **Radiographic Findings:** Bitewings 4 years ago, no other radiographs
Social History	Social drinker, 2 glasses of wine per week Patient reports excessive manual toothbrushing and flossing multiple times a day. Patient states she is afraid of developing caries. Parents have "bad teeth"	**Dental Findings:** Stable dentition

1. How would you educate this patient on homecare?
2. What manual technique of toothbrushing would you recommend? Why?
3. Would you recommend a power toothbrush? Why? What kind?
4. What other strategies would you implement?
5. What goals would you address?

25 Interdental and Supplemental Oral Self-Care Devices

COMPETENCIES

1. Relate the removal and control of interdental bacterial biofilm to current evidence regarding the prevention of oral disease.
2. Select effective self-care devices including interdental and supplemental self-care devices for each patient based on efficacy, individual client needs, and preferences. Also, discuss oral piercings and their impact on dental procedures, as well as the risks involved.
3. Educate patients as co-therapists in the safe and effective use of self-care devices designed for interdental and subgingival biofilm removal, considering oral conditions, patient preferences, risk factors present, and current evidence.

SHORT ANSWER QUESTIONS

1. List several tools used to assess clinical outcomes of biofilm removal effectiveness.

_____

_____

_____

_____

_____

2. List several considerations for interdental aid selection.

_____

_____

_____

_____

_____

_____

_____

_____

3. List several interdental devices to supplement biofilm removal in addition to toothbrushing.

_____

_____

_____

_____

_____

_____

_____

_____

4. What is the mechanism of action of a dental water jet?

_____

_____

_____

_____

5. What is the most common cause of halitosis?

_____

_____

_____

_____

6. List reasons why removing biofilm from areas where where a toothbrush does not reach is important.

_____

_____

_____

_____

VIDEO REVIEW QUESTIONS

The following questions are directed toward the Mechanical Oral Biofilm and Interdental Supplement videos located in Evolve. Watch the videos before answering the questions.

1. Under what conditions are interdental brushes to be used?

_____

_____

_____

_____

_____

_____

2. What are the functions of the rubber tip stimulator?

_____
_____
_____
_____
_____
_____

3. Under what conditions would a toothpick holder be used?

_____
_____
_____
_____

4. Under what conditions would a wooden wedge be indicated?

_____
_____
_____
_____
_____
_____

5. What are the indications for use of a floss threader?

_____
_____
_____
_____
_____

6. Floss holders are indicated for what type of patient?

_____
_____
_____
_____

7. Loop floss is indicated for what type of patient?

_____

_____

_____

_____

_____

_____

FILL IN THE BLANK STATEMENTS

Select the best term from the chapter and complete the following statements.

1. _____ is wider and flatter than traditional floss.

2. _____ has three distinct segments: floss, nylon mesh, and rigid plastic "needle."

3. _____ are plastic handles that aid in holding floss.

4. A device designed to assist with biofilm removal under fixed prosthetics, orthodontic bridges, and around abutments is the _____.

5. _____ that emit streams of water, reduce biofilm, bleeding, gingivitis, pocket depth, pathogenic microorganisms, and calculus.

6. Standard water jet tips can reach pocket depths up to _____ while specialty tips can reach periodontal; pockets up to _____.

MULTIPLE CHOICE QUESTIONS

Complete each question by circling the best answer.

1. Floss should be the first choice in interdental aids a patient uses to prevent and reverse gingival inflammation. Dental water jets are not as effective as floss for the reduction of interdental plaque biofilm, bleeding, and gingivitis.
   a. Both statements are true.
   b. Both statements are false.
   c. The first statement is true, the second statement is false.
   d. The first statement is false, the second statement is true.

2. There is no evidence supporting the effectiveness of an antimicrobial agent added to a dental water jet in a periodontal pocket. Specialty tips for dental water jets can allow >7 mm of solution into periodontal pockets.
   a. Both statements are true.
   b. Both statements are false.
   c. The first statement is true, the second statement is false.
   d. The first statement is false, the second statement is true.

3. The BEST choice for interdental biofilm removal in type II and type III embrasure spaces are:
   a. Dental tape
   b. Dental floss
   c. Rubber tip stimulator
   d. End-tufted toothbrush

4. Risks associated with oral piercings include all of the following EXCEPT:
   a. Gingivitis
   b. Recession
   c. Tooth fracture
   d. Bone loss

5. Since dental implants have no periodontal apparatus, they require very little plaque control and prevention interventions. The use of antimicrobial agents in dentifrices and mouthrinses is a good supplemental to daily toothbrushing for those patients with implants.
   a. Both statements are true.
   b. Both statements are false.
   c. The first statement is true, the second statement is false.
   d. The first statement is false, the second statement is true.

6. The spool method of flossing starts with all of the floss spooled on one finger of one hand, and as each new section is used, the used section is taken up and spooled on the other hand. The loop method of flossing ties the two ends of the floss together in a circle to move to a new section.
   a. Both statements are true.
   b. Both statements are false.
   c. The first statement is true, the second statement is false.
   d. The first statement is false, the second statement is true.

7. 'C' shape flossing should be used around mesial to distal interdental area. 'C' shape flossing is the easiest interdental device to suggest to patients.
   a. Both statements are true.
   b. Both statements are false.
   c. The first statement is true, the second statement is false.
   d. The first statement is false, the second statement is true.

CASE STUDY

Your 25-year-old patient reports for her 6-month recare appointment. She presents with slight biofilm generalized, slight calculus mandibular anterior, and pocket depths >3 mm generalized with slight bleeding interproximally on all molars. She reports using floss once a week but has difficulty reaching molars. She brushes once a day and demonstrates a scrubbing method of brushing.

1. What is her main unmet human need?
2. What is the etiology?
3. What are the signs and symptoms?
4. Develop attainable goals.
5. What is your education plan?

_____

_____

_____

_____

_____

_____

_____

_____

_____

26 Dentifrices

1. Explain the purpose of a dentifrice and the types of effects that it can produce.
2. Discuss the process of selecting the right dentifrice, including the role of dentifrices in the demineralization and remineralization process.
3. Describe the role of medicinal and nonmedicinal components in dentifrices.
4. Explain the concept of bioavailability.
5. Debate the possible adverse oral health effects of dentifrices.
6. Explain the impact of the pH level of dentifrices.
7. Analyze new trends in dentifrices (vegan, organic, etc.) and their potential effects on oral and global health.
8. Recommend dentifrices appropriate and their use for unique patient needs and risk factors.
9. Delineate the legal and ethical responsibilities of the DH with regard to dentifrices.

SHORT ANSWER QUESTIONS

1. Name seven agents present in most dentifrices.

_____

_____

_____

_____

_____

_____

_____

2. Name five therapeutic agent categories that may be present in a dentifrice.

_____

_____

_____

_____

_____

3. The demineralization threshold pH of cementum and dentin is:

_____

4. The demineralization threshold pH of enamel (hydroxyapatite) is:

_____

5. The demineralization threshold pH of fluorapatite enamel is:

_____

FILL IN THE BLANK STATEMENTS

Select the best term from the chapter and complete the following statements.

1. _____ is a broad-spectrum antimicrobial, anti-plaque, and anti-gingivitis agent found in some toothpastes.

2. _____ occurs when a medicinal agent is stable during storage and active when used to achieve the desired therapeutic effect.

3. _____ is tooth destruction caused by a substance harder than tooth structure.

4. _____ is cervical tooth structure destruction caused by excessive occlusal force.

5. _____ is tooth structure destruction resulting from excessive tooth-to-tooth friction.

6. _____ is tooth destruction as a result of a chemical agent.

7. An advantage of a higher abrasive dentifrice is _____.

8. A disadvantage of a higher abrasive dentifrice is _____.

MULTIPLE CHOICE QUESTIONS

Complete each question by circling the best answer.

1. A dentifrice assists patients achieve all of the following effects EXCEPT:
   a. Hygienic
   b. Therapeutic
   c. Restorative
   d. Cosmetic

2. A dentifrice that does not have the ADA seal of approval is unsafe for patient use. Dental hygienists should only recommend dentifrices with the ADA seal of approval.
   a. Both statements are true.
   b. Both statements are false.
   c. The first statement is true, the second statement is false.
   d. The first statement is false, the second statement is true.

3. There is no scientific evidence to support the effectiveness of:
   a. Activated charcoal as a whitening agent
   b. Stannous fluoride as an anti-calculus agent
   c. Chlorhexidine gluconate to control oral biofilm formation
   d. Tricoslan as an antibacterial additive.

4. The best dentifrice recommendation for a patient with severe recession is:
   a. Low abrasiveness
   b. Low pH
   c. Added sodium bicarbonate
   d. Added charcoal

5. All of the following health conditions should be considered when recommending a dentifrice EXCEPT:
   a. Substance intolerance
   b. Allergies
   c. Kidney disease
   d. Hypertension

6. If abrasive capacity of a dentifrice is too low, soft deposits and stains will not be removed adequately. If abrasive capacity if a dentifrice is too high, it may abraid natural and restored tooth structures.
   a. Both statements are true.
   b. Both statements are false.
   c. The first statement is true, the second statement is false.
   d. The first statement is false, the second statement is true.

7. A dentifrice can prevent an oral disease when it provides a therapeutic function. A dentifrice can be a risk factor for causing dentin hypersensitivity, erosion, or abrasion.
   a. Both statements are true.
   b. Both statements are false.
   c. The first statement is true, the second statement is false.
   d. The first statement is false, the second statement is true.

8. The desensitizing agent that creates a chemical action is:
   a. Xylitol
   b. Aluminum
   c. Calcium
   d. Potassium nitrate

9. The desensitizing agent that creates a mechanical action includes all of the following EXCEPT:
   a. Sodium fluoride
   b. Stannous fluoride
   c. Recaldent
   d. Potassium chloride

10. Your patient reports moderate sensitivity to cold and pressure when brushing receded areas. Recommending a desensitizing toothpaste satisfies which Human Needs deficit?
    a. Protection from Health Risks
    b. Wholesome Facial Image
    c. Freedom from Pain
    d. Responsibility for Oral Health

11. Which nanoparticle found in oral health products should pregnant women avoid?
    a. Titanium dioxide
    b. Hydrogen peroxide
    c. Sodium bicarbonate
    d. Stannous fluoride

Your 15-year-old female patient presents to your office for routine dental hygiene care. Initial observations are:

- Thin, frail body type
- Pale skin, dark circles under eyes
- Quiet demeanor

Extra/intraoral exam findings:

- High caries rate
- Slight biofilm
- Very slight calculus
- Moderate erosion on all lingual tooth surfaces
- Erythematous shiny tissue on palatal tissues
- Periodontal probe readings are >3 mm generalized.

Patient reports severe tooth sensitivity. She states she brushes once a day with a whitening toothpaste. She also uses a charcoal toothpaste she ordered from the internet. She says flossing hurts. She also states that she would like to whiten her teeth with in-office whitening gel.

1. What possible conclusion could you draw from your clinical findings?
2. What dietary recommendations will you make?
3. What dentifrice will you recommend? Why?
4. What Human Needs Model deficits does this patient have?

_____

_____

_____

_____

_____

_____

_____

_____

_____

_____

_____

_____

_____

_____

_____

_____

27 Antimicrobial Agents for Control of Periodontal Disease

COMPETENCIES

1. Outline the mechanisms for ensuring efficacy, quality, and safety of periodontal antimicrobial products.
2. Explain the rationale for adjunctive antimicrobial biofilm control.
3. Compare and contrast delivery methods of antimicrobial agents for both home and professional use.
4. Discuss the evidence regarding effectiveness of various active ingredients included in antimicrobial products for the treatment of periodontal diseases.
5. Apply evidence-based indications for use of antimicrobial agents as interventions for the prevention and treatment of periodontal diseases.

SHORT ANSWER QUESTIONS

1. What is an active ingredient in an antimicrobial agent?

_____

_____

_____

_____

2. List the criteria for ADA Seal of Acceptance for antimicrobial non-prescription therapeutic mouthrinses.

_____

_____

_____

_____

_____

3. What are the therapeutic effects of mouthrinses with essential oils?

_____

_____

_____

_____

_____

_____

_____

_____

_____

_____

_____

4. List the patients who should not use alcohol-based mouthrinses.

_____

_____

_____

_____

_____

_____

_____

_____

_____

5. Briefly describe the benefit of lasers in dentistry.

_____

_____

_____

_____

_____

6. List recommended properties of an oral rinse.

_____

_____

_____

_____

_____

_____

_____

_____

_____

_____

_____

VIDEO REVIEW QUESTIONS

The following questions are directed toward the antimicrobials videos located on Evolve. Watch the following videos and answer the questions:

- Placing Controlled-Release Drug: Doxycycline Gel
- Placing Controlled-Release Drug: Minocycline Hydrochloride Microspheres

1. What is the percentage of doxycycline hyclate gel used in the video?

_____

_____

2. How long is the controlled release for a Chlorhexidine Chip?

_____

_____

3. What are the clinical indications for using doxycycline hyclate gel?

_____

_____

_____

_____

4. Minocycline hydrochloride microspheres is also known as:

_____

_____

5. When is minocycline hydrochloride microspheres indicated for use?

_____

_____

FILL IN THE BLANK STATEMENTS

Select the best term from the chapter and complete the following statements.

1. _____ use an active agent within a delivery system to prevent or control periodontal disease.

2. _____ are also known as chemotherapeutic agents.

3. _____ is the ability of a therapeutic agent to be retained and released over time to increase effectiveness.

4. _____ uses a sub-antimicrobial system dose for purposes other than destruction of pathogenic microorganisms.

5. _____ is an intervention is used by itself.

6. Live microorganisms that have health benefits for the host when administered alone or in combination is considered _____

7. Powered and manual devices that deliver an active ingredient within a solution via an irrigation tip into the gingival sulcus or periodontal pocket is a(n) _____

MULTIPLE CHOICE QUESTIONS

Complete each question by circling the best answer.

1. What federal government agency determines safe and effective products such as oral antimicrobial agents?
   a. CDC
   b. FDA
   c. ADA
   d. USDA

2. What is a common side effect of chlorhexidine gluconate oral rinses?
   a. Gingival ulcerations
   b. Enamel stain
   c. Burning tongue syndrome
   d. Excess salivation

3. Which statement most closely describes sub-antimicrobial systemic dose of antibiotics?
   a. Prescribed for patients with uncontrolled diabetes
   b. Loading dose of the medication is all that is needed
   c. Administrated for short-term periodontal therapy
   d. Use of medication at a reduced dose for alternative use

4. Which of the following antimicrobial agents has the highest recommendation?
   a. Chlorhexidine chip
   b. Doxycycline hyclate
   c. Atridox
   d. Minocycline microsphere

5. Which of the following laser therapies is ADA recommended?
   a. Nd-YAG
   b. Photodynamic therapy diode
   c. Non-PDT diode
   d. CO_2

6. Which entity guides practitioners and patients on the safety and efficacy of oral health products?
   a. CDA
   b. FDA
   c. NDA
   d. ADA

7. Local delivery of an antimicrobial agent is applied directly to a specific location in the oral cavity. Systemic delivery of an antimicrobial agent is a medication that are ingested by the patient and delivered via the bloodstream.
   a. Both statements are true.
   b. Both statements are false.
   c. The first statement is true, the second statement is false.
   d. The first statement is false, the second statement is true.

8. Bacteriostatic means that microbes are destroyed directly whereas bactericidal means the metabolism or reproduction of the microbe is disrupted.
   a. Both statements are true.
   b. Both statements are false.
   c. The first statement is true, the second statement is false.
   d. The first statement is false, the second statement is true.

9. What is not a side effect of chlorhexidine gluconate oral rinse?
   a. Staining
   b. Taste alteration
   c. Increased calculus accumulation
   d. Gingival sloughing

10. Which of the following statement is not true concerning chlorhexidine gluconate oral rinse?
    a. Usual recommendation is to rinse for 1 minute twice a day
    b. After CHX use, wait to rinse with water for 30 minutes
    c. After CHX use, wait to brush with toothpaste for 30 minutes
    d. After CHX use, wait to eat hot or sticky foods for 30 minutes

11. An agent's ability to durably bind with oral tissues and then be released over a period of time, aiding in a product's effectiveness is:
    a. Substantivity
    b. Bactericidal
    c. Bacteriostatic
    d. Antiseptic

12. Cetylpyridium chloride-based mouthrinses have antimicrobial properties. Cetylpyridium chloride-based mouthrinses have clinically significant plaque and gingivitis reductions as demonstrated in long-term clinical trials.
    a. Both statements are true.
    b. Both statements are false.
    c. The first statement is true, the second statement is false.
    d. The first statement is false, the second statement is true.

13. The lowest concentration of a particular antimicrobial that is able to inhibit microbial growth during incubation is:
    a. Controlled release drug delivery
    b. Minimum inhibitory concentration
    c. Minimum clinical effectiveness
    d. Controlled inhibitory concentration

14. Which of the following is an example of a home-use local antimicrobial agent?
    a. Chlorhexidine chip
    b. Listerine mouth rinse
    c. Prescription fluoride
    d. Minocycline microspheres

15. All of the following are true concerning the systemic delivery of antibiotics for the treatment of periodontal disease EXCEPT:
    a. Low concentrations of antibiotics are delivered to diseased sites
    b. Recommended to treat persistent periodontitis
    c. Antibiotic reaches infected sites through the blood stream then through gingival crevicular fluid
    d. Antibiotic can reach multiple sites at the same time

Performance Objective

By following a routine procedure that meets the stated protocols, the student will demonstrate the appropriate technique for **27.1 Placement of controlled release drug: CHX chip**

Evaluation and Grading Criteria

Instructor will assign grades for each performance criteria.

3 Student competently met stated criteria
2 Student required minimal assistance to meet criteria
1 Student showed uncertainty when attempting criteria
0 Student was not prepared and needs to repeat criteria
N/A Student was not evaluated

Performance Standards

Instructor shall identify steps that are critical with an asterisk (*)

Performance Criteria	*	Self	Peer	Instructor	Comments
1. Equipment Personal protective equipment Mouth mirror Periodontal probe Cotton pliers, cotton rolls, dry angles Scaler(s) Chlorhexidine chips					
2. Determine need for controlled-release chlorhexidine chip therapy; explain risks and benefits and alternatives to treatment. Obtain informed consent.					
3. Review medical and oral history; evaluate contraindications to and precautions for treatment.					
4. Remove required number of chips from package; note that product is stored at controlled room temperature of 59° to 77°F (15° to 25°C).					
5. Isolate and dry area to prevent wetting chip during placement; grasp square end of chip with cotton pliers, and insert subgingivally.					
6. Use cotton pliers or an instrument of choice to insert chip into deepest part of pocket.					
7. Instruct the client as a co-therapist not to floss area for 10 days and inform him or her that some moderate sensitivity may be experienced for about 1 week in the area of placement. Client should clean other areas of mouth as usual and call the office if any pain, swelling, or problem occurs.					

Continued

Performance Criteria	*	Self	Peer	Instructor	Comments
8. Schedule reevaluation and/or reapplication. Reevaluation of probe depths and clinical attachment levels can coincide with periodontal maintenance visit.					
9. Document the intervention in detail in patient's record under services provided and date the entry; include tooth numbers and sites and post-operative instructions given.					
10. Prevention of Disease Transmission	*				
ADDITIONAL COMMENTS					

28 Hand-Activated Instrumentation

COMPETENCIES

1. Discuss the functional components of hand-activated instruments used in nonsurgical periodontal care.
2. Differentiate periodontal treatment and assessment hand-activated instruments.
3. Select design considerations for assessment and treatment instruments based on the periodontal health status and needs of a patient.
4. Relate the basic stroke principles of hand-activated instrumentation to the requirements for effective instrumentation.
5. Discuss treatment instrument selection and criteria considerations in determining the appropriate instrument design and blade size and customize details regarding their sequencing and use for periodontitis-affected teeth.
6. Elucidate the benefits and ethical principles associated with maintaining sharp hand-activated instruments.
7. Describe the application of basic elements of instrumentation skills to optimize effective treatment and minimize risk for injury.
8. Summarize the key elements of comprehensive post-treatment patient education.

SHORT ANSWER QUESTIONS

1. What is the terminal shank to the end of the instrument called?

_____

_____

2. List and identify the working end designs of a universal instrument.

_____

_____

_____

_____

_____

3. List the considerations when selecting an instrument.

_____

_____

_____

_____

_____

_____

_____

_____

4. List the uses for the periodontal probe.

_____

_____

_____

_____

_____

_____

_____

_____

_____

_____

5. List the positive aspects of sharp instruments and the negative aspects of dull instruments.

_____

_____

_____

_____

_____

_____

_____

_____

_____

6. List expectations a patient may experience after periodontal treatment.

_____

_____

_____

_____

_____

_____

_____

_____

_____

_____

VIDEO REVIEW QUESTIONS

The following questions are directed toward the hand-activated instrument videos located on Evolve. Watch the videos and answer the questions.

1. When are Gracey curettes indicated for use?
   a. For patients with slight to severe periodontal disease
   b. For patients who require scaling and root debriding

   _____
   _____
   _____
   _____
   _____
   _____

2. What is the angulation degree range for Gracey curettes?

   _____
   _____
   _____

3. Which Gracey curette is most appropriate for instrumenting the mesial surface of tooth no. 3?

   _____
   _____
   _____
   _____

4. Which Gracey curette is most appropriate for instrumenting the distal surface of tooth no. 19?

   _____
   _____
   _____
   _____

5. Which Gracey curette is most appropriate for instrumenting the distal surface of tooth no. 9?

   _____
   _____
   _____
   _____

6. Rigid Graceys are most appropriate for which periodontal conditions?

   _____
   _____
   _____
   _____

7. Standard Graceys are most appropriate for which periodontal conditions?

   _____
   _____
   _____
   _____

149

8. How is the After Five Gracey design different from standard and rigid designs?

_____

_____

_____

9. How is the Mini Five Gracey design different from standard and rigid designs?

_____

_____

_____

10. Sickle scalers with straight shanks are designed for which teeth?

_____

_____

_____

11. Tissue allowing, how deep can a sickle scaler go subgingivally safely?

_____

_____

_____

12. On what teeth and surfaces can posterior sickle scalers be used to scale calculus?

_____

_____

_____

13. Do sickle scalers have a rounded toe or a pointed tip?

_____

_____

_____

14. Where is the S204S is best used?

_____

_____

_____

15. Are universal curettes used supragingivally or subgingivally?

_____

_____

_____

16. Do universal curettes have a rounded toe or a pointed tip?

_____

_____

_____

17. What are common instrument designs of universal curettes?

_____

_____

_____

_____

_____

18. What blade angle of universal curette is ideal for insertion into a pocket?

_____

_____

_____

19. What blade angle of universal curette is ideal for calculus removal in a pocket?

_____

_____

_____

20. Is the angulation and activation of a universal blade set at 45 degrees adequate for effective calculus removal? Why or why not?

_____

_____

_____

21. Is the angulation and activation of a universal blade set at 90 degrees adequate for effective calculus removal? Why or why not?

_____

_____

_____

FILL IN THE BLANK STATEMENTS

Select the best term from the chapter and complete the following statements.

1. The _____ is the inclusive total shank that includes a bend nearest to the handle to the tip of the working end.

2. The _____ is within the functional shank that includes the last bend to the working end.

3. A shank that is _____ is best for pockets with deep probing depths or recession.

4. Instruments that have short shanks and fewer bends are best suited for _____ teeth.

5. Instruments that have long shanks and more bends are best suited for _____ teeth.

Complete each question by circling the best answer.

1. Flexible shanks are used for detecting and removing light calculus or biofilm. Moderate flexible shanks are best for removing moderate calculus deposits.
   a. Both statements are true.
   b. Both statements are false.
   c. The first statement is true, the second statement is false.
   d. The first statement is false, the second statement is true.

2. All of the following are components to test for instrument sharpness EXCEPT:
   a. Auditory
   b. Tactile
   c. Strength
   d. Visual

3. Which grasp is recommended when holding an instrument for sharpening?
   a. Pen Grasp
   b. Modified Pen Grasp
   c. Extended Modified Pen Grasp
   d. Palm-Thumb Grasp

4. All of the following are assessment instruments EXCEPT:
   a. 11/12 explorer
   b. Periodontal probe
   c. 1/2 gracey
   d. Mouth mirror

5. Which instrument is the BEST choice for debriding slight soft and hard deposits in a healthy periodontium during routine oral hygiene care?
   a. Universal curet
   b. Gracey curet
   c. 11/12 explorer
   d. Sickle scaler

6. All of the following are uses of the mouth mirror EXCEPT:
   a. Direct vision
   b. Transillumination
   c. Retraction
   d. Indirect illumination

7. All of the following are types of instrument strokes EXCEPT:
   a. Root planing
   b. Angulation
   c. Scaling
   d. Exploratory

8. Which Gracey has a 50% reduced blade as compared to the traditional Gracey curet?
   a. Slim line
   b. Extended
   c. Mini bladed
   d. Micro bladed

9. Which instrument is the BEST choice for removing heavy supragingival calculus of mandibular anterior teeth?
   a. Universal curet
   b. Gracey curet
   c. 11/12 explorer
   d. Sickle scaler

10. Your patient presents with moderate burnished calculus subgingivally on all posterior teeth. What is the BEST choice for roughening the burnished areas of calculus?
    a. Sickle scaler
    b. Standard Gracey curet
    c. Universal curet
    d. Hirschfeld files

11. Which instrument would NOT be recommended to remove slight to moderate calculus in pocket depths of 5-6 mm on maxillary second molars?
    a. Sickle scaler
    b. Standard Gracey curet
    c. Universal curet
    d. Hirschfeld files

12. The 1N Nabors probe is only used for the detection and classification of mesial and distal furcations of maxillary molars. The 2N Nabors probe is only used for the detection and classification of buccal and lingual furcations.
    a. Both statements are true.
    b. Both statements are false
    c. The first statement is true, the second statement is false.
    d. The first statement is false, the second statement is true.

CASE STUDY

Your patient presents for scale and root debridement of maxillary right quadrant. All teeth are present in the quadrant. Molars have class I furcation. Probe readings are generalized 5-7 mm generalized with 1-2 mm recession generalized. Taking into account furcations, recession, and periodontal pocket measurements, develop a plan for generalized moderate calculus removal and root debridement. Identify which instruments are most appropriate for each sextant/tooth and why.

Performance Objective

By following a routine procedure that meets the stated protocols, the student will demonstrate the appropriate technique for **PROCEDURE 28.1 USE OF ASSESSMENT INSTRUMENTS: Periodontal Probe**

Evaluation and Grading Criteria

Instructor will assign grades for each performance criteria.

<u>3</u> Student competently met stated criteria
<u>2</u> Student required minimal assistance to meet criteria
<u>1</u> Student showed uncertainty when attempting criteria
<u>0</u> Student was not prepared and needs to repeat criteria
<u>N/A</u> Student was not evaluated

Performance Standards

Instructor shall identify steps that are critical with an asterisk (*)

Performance Criteria	*	Self	Peer	Instructor	Comments
1. Equipment Periodontal Probe Mouth mirror					
2. Grasp Type- Pen or Modified Pen Pressure - Light grasp; increase when discerning tooth structure, restorative materials, calculus					
3. Fulcrum and Pressure Pressure - Relatively light and adjustable Placement - Intraoral, adjacent to tooth being instrumented, cross-arch, opposite arch, extraoral					
4. Working End Selection Periodontal probe - Typically one working end however can be on one end of unpaired instrument					
5. Insertion, Adaptation, Angulation **Periodontal Probe** Insertion – Working end parallel to long axis of tooth until the junctional epithelium is contacted Adaptation – Keep lower 1 to 3 mm of probe against tooth Angulation – Angle tip area directly under contact (col) at the interproximal area, with shank touching the contact **Furcation Probe** Insertion - Select side of working end that fits parallel and 0° to the long axis of the tooth, not perpendicular. Guided by radiographs, previously recorded probing depths, and root anatomy knowledge, negotiate furcation probe into the area of the suspected furcation Adaptation – Gently rotate the probe tip toward the entrance of the furcation and note extent of penetration and classification **Implant Probe** Insertion – Gently insert into the peri-implant sulcus until slight resistance is met. Maintain light pressure to avoid penetration of the implant mucosal attachment Adaptation – Adapt implant probe to implant surface					

Continued

153

Performance Criteria	*	Self	Peer	Instructor	Comments
6. Activation Walk probe with gentle pressure along base of sulcus or pocket where the junctional epithelium feels soft and resilient; maintain one side of probe in contact with tooth surface					
7. Stroke Direction Small, vertical increments					
8. Efficiency Insert toward distal of tooth; walk distally in small 1 mm increments until distal col area (under contact) of tooth is reached with upper portion of probe straightened and touching contact area Lift probe and reinsert at distal line angle; repeat technique by walking forward to mesial col area Continue throughout mouth buccally and lingually to six deepest readings of distal, buccal or lingual, and mesial surfaces from both buccal and lingual approach					
9. Prevention of Disease Transmission	*				
ADDITIONAL COMMENTS					

Performance Objective

By following a routine procedure that meets the stated protocols, the student will demonstrate the appropriate technique for **PROCEDURE 28.1 USE OF ASSESSMENT INSTRUMENTS: Periodontal Explorer**

Evaluation and Grading Criteria

Instructor will assign grades for each performance criteria.

<u>3</u> Student competently met stated criteria
<u>2</u> Student required minimal assistance to meet criteria
<u>1</u> Student showed uncertainty when attempting criteria
<u>0</u> Student was not prepared and needs to repeat criteria
<u>N/A</u> Student was not evaluated

Performance Standards

Instructor shall identify steps that are critical with an asterisk (*)

Performance Criteria	*	Self	Peer	Instructor	Comments
1. Equipment Periodontal explorer Mouth mirror					
2. Grasp Type- Pen or Modified Pen Pressure - Light to moderate grasp; increase when discerning tooth structure, restorative materials, calculus					
3. Fulcrum and Pressure Pressure - Relatively light/moderate Placement - Intraoral, adjacent to tooth being instrumented, cross-arch, opposite arch, extraoral					
4. Working End Selection 3-A explorer: Typically one working end 11/12 explorer (extended for deep periodontal pockets): Paired with two working ends.					
5. Insertion Insertion - insert with lower end of explorer curved toward tooth until the junctional epithelium is contacted Adaptation: Lower 1-3 mm of explorer tip touching root surface					
6. Adaptation Lower 1-3 mm of explorer tip touching root surface					
7. Activation Begin activation with insertion stroke (vertical) with both a push-and-pull stroke Light pressure: friable tissue, light calculus, final assessment Increased pressure: root irregularities, moderate to heavy calculus, burnished calculus					
Stroke Direction Multidirectional strokes to assess calculus, burnished deposits, root caries or restorative margins; upward and downward direction for detecting burnished or sheet-like calculus					

Continued

155

Performance Criteria	*	Self	Peer	Instructor	Comments
8. Efficiency Long and sweeping strokes: Evaluate root smoothness **Short** strokes: Encountering pieces of calculus or surface irregularities					
9. Prevention of Disease Transmission	*				
ADDITIONAL COMMENTS					

COMPETENCY CHAPTER 28 HAND-ACTIVATED INSTRUMENTATION

Performance Objective

By following a routine procedure that meets the stated protocols, the student will demonstrate the appropriate technique for **PROCEDURE 28.2 USE OF CURETS: Universal Curet**

Evaluation and Grading Criteria

Instructor will assign grades for each performance criteria.

<u>3</u> Student competently met stated criteria
<u>2</u> Student required minimal assistance to meet criteria
<u>1</u> Student showed uncertainty when attempting criteria
<u>0</u> Student was not prepared and needs to repeat criteria
<u>N/A</u> Student was not evaluated

Performance Standards

Instructor shall identify steps that are critical with an asterisk (*)

Performance Criteria	*	Self	Peer	Instructor	Comments
1. Equipment Universal Curet					
2. Grasp Type - Modified Pen Pressure - Secure; responsive to changes by allowing handle (hence blade) to fluidly roll during calculus removal and around root topography such as line angles, convexities, and concavities					
3. Fulcrum and Pressure Pressure - Stable, moderate with working stroke; increases with tenacity of calculus Placement - Intraoral, adjacent to tooth being scaled Cross-arch, opposite arch, extraoral					
4. Working End Selection Posterior - Position universal blade against buccal or lingual surface of tooth and choose end that offers a more closed adaptation Anterior - Either working end					
5. Insertion Blade in relatively closed position to base of pocket (0-10°)					
6. Adaptation Adjust first 2 to 3 mm of blade against tooth surface using tactile sensations					
7. Angulation Open blade to between 60 and 80 degrees					
8. Activation Re-secure grasp and fulcrum to achieve an effective working stroke; modify pressure against tooth by type, amount and position of calculus and/or tooth irregularity; utilization of the proper fingers to maximize lateral pressure and fluid strokes					

Continued

157

Copyright © 2025 by Elsevier Inc. All rights are reserved, including those for text and data mining, AI training, and similar technologies.

Chapter **28** **Hand-Activated Instrumentation**

Performance Criteria	*	Self	Peer	Instructor	Comments
9. Stroke Direction Vertical, horizontal, and oblique pull stroke; vary stroke directions to complete calculus removal/root planing					
Implant Considerations Other professional methods for biofilm removal: subgingival glycine air polishing Implant universal curet: thin, mini-bladed or longer blade if access is needed around restorations Healthy: gentle sweeping, nonaggressive strokes Mucositis: short horizontal strokes, overlapping and/or vertical if accessible and adaptable Peri-implantitis and Failing: thin blade used in slight side-to-side movements to debride around implant threads and refer					
10. Prevention of Disease Transmission	*				
ADDITIONAL COMMENTS					

Performance Objective

By following a routine procedure that meets the stated protocols, the student will demonstrate the appropriate technique for **PROCEDURE 28.2 USE OF CURETS: Area-Specific Curet**

Evaluation and Grading Criteria

Instructor will assign grades for each performance criteria.

3 Student competently met stated criteria
2 Student required minimal assistance to meet criteria
1 Student showed uncertainty when attempting criteria
0 Student was not prepared and needs to repeat criteria
N/A Student was not evaluated

Performance Standards

Instructor shall identify steps that are critical with an asterisk (*)

Performance Criteria	*	Self	Peer	Instructor	Comments
1. Equipment Area-specific curet					
2. Grasp Type - modified pen Pressure - Secure; responsive to changes by allowing handle (hence blade) to fluidly roll during calculus removal and around root topography such as line angles, convexities, and concavities					
3. Fulcrum and Pressure Pressure - Stable, moderate with working stroke; increases with tenacity of calculus Placement - Intraoral, adjacent to tooth being scaled Cross-arch, opposite arch, extraoral					
4. Working End Selection Position longer, lower cutting edge of offset blade against tooth; for vertical stroke, face of blade toward root surface, lower shank is parallel to the long axis of the tooth or root surface being scaled					
5. Insertion: Blade in relatively closed position to base of pocket (0-10°)					
6. Adaptation Adjust first 2 to 3 mm of blade against tooth surface using tactile sensations					
7. Angulation Open blade to between 60 and 80 degrees					
8. Activation Re-secure grasp and fulcrum to achieve an effective working stroke; modify pressure against tooth by type, amount and position of calculus and/or tooth irregularity; utilization of the proper fingers to maximize lateral pressure and fluid strokes					

Continued

Performance Criteria	*	Self	Peer	Instructor	Comments
9. Stroke Direction Vertical, horizontal, oblique pull stroke; vary stroke directions to complete calculus removal/root planing					
10. Implant Considerations Other professional methods for biofilm removal: subgingival glycine air polishing Implant area-specific set: thin, mini- or micro-bladed with longer angled shanks if access is needed around restorations Healthy: gentle sweeping, non-aggressive strokes Mucositis: short horizontal strokes, overlapping and/or vertical if accessible and adaptable Peri-implantitis and Failing: thin, small blade used in slight side-to-side movements to debride around implant threads and refer					
11. Prevention of Disease Transmission	*				
ADDITIONAL COMMENTS					

Performance Objective

By following a routine procedure that meets the stated protocols, the student will demonstrate the appropriate technique for **PROCEDURE 28.3 USE OF SICKLE SCALERS: Posterior Sickle**

Evaluation and Grading Criteria

Instructor will assign grades for each performance criteria.

<u>3</u> Student competently met stated criteria
<u>2</u> Student required minimal assistance to meet criteria
<u>1</u> Student showed uncertainty when attempting criteria
<u>0</u> Student was not prepared and needs to repeat criteria
<u>N/A</u> Student was not evaluated

Performance Standards

Instructor shall identify steps that are critical with an asterisk (*)

Performance Criteria	*	Self	Peer	Instructor	Comments
1. Equipment Posterior sickle					
2. Grasp Type - Modified Pen Pressure - Moderate grasp					
3. Fulcrum and Pressure Pressure - Stable and moderate Placement - Intraoral, adjacent to tooth being scaled, opposite arch					
4. Working End Selection Based on amount of calculus, tissue tone, pocket depth, and correct adaptation; location can influence blade size					
5. Insertion Use opposite end for alternate sides of tooth. Engage lower edge of interproximal supragingival calculus however may extend 1 to 2 mm subgingivally when soft tissue permits					
6. Adaptation Lower third cutting edge and tip of sickle closely adapted to tooth surface Engage lower edge of supragingival calculus Engage ledge of subgingival calculus by keeping side of tip well adapted to root surface					
7. Angulation Adjust blade to 80 to 90 degrees against tooth surface					
8. Activation, Stroke and Direction <u>Supragingival:</u> Vertical to oblique pull stroke with moderate pressure across tooth surface <u>Subgingival:</u> Vertical pull stroke using moderate pressure across subgingival area					

Continued

161

Performance Criteria	*	Self	Peer	Instructor	Comments
9. **Efficiency** Repeat until all gross calculus is removed					
10. Prevention of Disease Transmission	*				
ADDITIONAL COMMENTS					

Performance Objective

By following a routine procedure that meets the stated protocols, the student will demonstrate the appropriate technique for **PROCEDURE 28.3 USE OF SICKLE SCALERS: Anterior Sickle**

Evaluation and Grading Criteria

Instructor will assign grades for each performance criteria.

3 Student competently met stated criteria
2 Student required minimal assistance to meet criteria
1 Student showed uncertainty when attempting criteria
0 Student was not prepared and needs to repeat criteria
N/A Student was not evaluated

Performance Standards

Instructor shall identify steps that are critical with an asterisk (*)

Performance Criteria	*	Self	Peer	Instructor	Comments
1. Equipment Anterior sickle					
2. Grasp Type- modified pen Pressure – moderate grasp					
3. Fulcrum and Pressure Pressure - Stable and moderate Placement - Intraoral, adjacent to tooth being scaled, opposite arch					
4. Working End Selection Based on amount of calculus, tissue tone, pocket depth, and correct adaptation Thinner-tip designed sickles can be used for calculus located just below tight, anterior contacts areas					
Insertion Engage lower edge of interproximal supragingival calculus; however, may extend 1 to 2 mm subgingivally when soft tissue permits					
5. Adaptation Lower third cutting edge and tip of sickle closely adapted to tooth surface					
6. Angulation Adjust blade to 80 to 90 degrees against tooth surface					
Activation, Stroke and Direction Supragingival: Vertical to oblique pull stroke with moderate pressure across tooth surface Subgingival: Vertical pull stroke using moderate pressure across subgingival area					

Continued

Performance Criteria	*	Self	Peer	Instructor	Comments
7. Efficiency Repeat until all gross calculus is removed					
8. Prevention of Disease Transmission	*				
ADDITIONAL COMMENTS					

29 Ultrasonic Instrumentation

COMPETENCIES

1. Value the role of ultrasonic instrumentation in accomplishing the objectives of periodontal debridement in terms of the advantages and indications.
2. Relate the mechanisms of action of ultrasonic instruments to effective debridement of the tooth/root surface.
3. Compare and contrast magnetostrictive and piezoelectric ultrasonic scaling instruments.
4. Discuss the acoustic power produced by an ultrasonic scaler.
5. Apply information about the relationship of key operational and technique variables to the mechanisms of ultrasonic debridement.
   - Produce a level of acoustic power suitable for the treatment objective through proper adjustment of the operational variables.
   - Consider the influence of tip design on clinical performance to guide tip selection based on the treatment objective and the anatomy of the treatment site.
6. Execute proper ultrasonic instrumentation technique with any tip design in any area of the dentition.
7. Discuss assessment and management of using ultrasonic instrumentation for patient care.

SHORT ANSWER QUESTIONS

1. What mechanisms of action are used to disrupt tooth surface deposits during ultrasonic instrumentation?

_____

_____

_____

_____

2. The human ear hears below what frequency?

_____

_____

_____

3. Briefly describe the method of action in ultrasonic scaling.

_____

_____

_____

_____

_____

_____

4. How is an ultrasonic tip selected?

_____

_____

_____

_____

_____

5. Explain the working stroke during ultrasonic instrumentation.

_____

_____

_____

_____

_____

6. Describe strategies that allow for most efficiently implementing instrumentation.

_____

_____

_____

_____

_____

_____

7. List strategies to minimize aerosol cross-contamination.

_____

_____

_____

_____

_____

8. List and describe designs of ultrasonic tips.

_____

_____

_____

_____

_____

9. Which ultrasonic tips are most appropriate for removing biofilm or light calculus?

_____

_____

_____

_____

_____

_____

_____

_____

_____

_____

_____

10. List the objectives of root surface debridement.

_____

_____

_____

_____

_____

FILL IN THE BLANK STATEMENTS

Select the best term from the chapter and complete the following statements.

1. Forward and backward movement of an ultrasonic tip at high frequency is called _____.

2. Fluid flow generated by ultrasonic oscillations is _____.

3. The number of complete back and forth strokes the oscillating tip completes per second, measured in kilohertz (kHz) is called the _____.

4. _____, or stroke length, is measured as how far the tip is displaced from a position of zero movement.

5. A standard rectangular ultrasonic tip with two bends is most appropriate to remove _____.

6. The overall goal of periodontal debridement is _____.

MULTIPLE CHOICE QUESTIONS

Complete each question by circling the best answer.

1. Cavitation and acoustic microstreaming are generated by the vibrating tip transmitting ultrasonic energy into the irrigating water. Cavitation and acoustic microstreaming are hydrodynamic forces capable of disrupting plaque biofilm.
   a. Both statements are true.
   b. Both statements are false.
   c. The first statement is true, the second statement is false.
   d. The first statement is false, the second statement is true.

2. To set adequate flow rate, water flow rate, adjust the water flow control until droplets are released from the tip at a low power setting. A flow rate of 20-30 ml/min provides an adequate supply of water for cooling as well as cavitation/microstreaming.
   a. Both statements are true.
   b. Both statements are false.
   c. The first statement is true, the second statement is false.
   d. The first statement is false, the second statement is true.

167

3. The operating frequency of an ultrasonic scaler has very little significance. Tip diameter and shape have a direct impact on mechanisms of action.
   a. Both statements are true.
   b. Both statements are false.
   c. The first statement is true, the second statement is false.
   d. The first statement is false, the second statement is true.

4. To accomplish efficient deposit removal without over-instrumentation of the root surface, the ultrasonic scaler should be used at the maximum effective acoustic power level. The minimum level of acoustic power needed will vary according to the type of deposit to be removed.
   a. Both statements are true.
   b. Both statements are false.
   c. The first statement is true, the second statement is false.
   d. The first statement is false, the second statement is true.

5. The ultrasonic tip diameter that has the greater mass is:
   a. Slim
   b. Ultra-slim
   c. Standard
   d. Fine

6. Vibrations produce microscopic high- and low-pressure areas that form bubbles filled with water vapor rather than air. The vibration stretches and compresses tiny bubbles until they implode and release a burst of heat and pressure. This action is called:
   a. Oscillation
   b. Acoustic microstreaming
   c. Cavitation
   d. Ultrasonic

7. A magnetostrictive ultrasonic scaler includes an insert composed of a stack of thin metal strips soldered together at the ends and attached by a connecting body to a tip. The handpiece contains a crystalline disk that expands and contracts in response to electrical current.
   a. Both statements are true.
   b. Both statements are false.
   c. The first statement is true, the second statement is false.
   d. The first statement is false, the second statement is true.

8. An increase in power will increase the displacement amplitude. A decrease in power will decrease the displacement amplitude.
   a. Both statements are true.
   b. Both statements are false.
   c. The first statement is true, the second statement is false.
   d. The first statement is false, the second statement is true.

9. The net force exerted by the oscillating tip directly correlates to the tip's diameter and to the displacement amplitude. The circular-shaped tip exerts greater force compared to a rectangular-shaped tip.
   a. Both statements are true.
   b. Both statements are false.
   c. The first statement is true, the second statement is false.
   d. The first statement is false, the second statement is true.

10. Which type of tip is to only be used during open flap periodontal surgery?
    a. Carbon fiber
    b. Plastic
    c. Diamond
    d. Nickel

11. The most common tip adaptation to tooth using any ultrasonic device is:
    a. Horizontal
    b. Vertical
    c. Oblique
    d. Cross hatch

12. Opening the active area of the oscillating tip more than 15-degree angulation:
    a. Is standard contact of tip to tooth
    b. Negatively alters root surfaces
    c. Is better for hard deposit removal
    d. Requires applying more lateral pressure

13. The ultra-slim tip is available in what shape(s)?
    a. Rectangle
    b. Triangle
    c. Circular
    d. Circular and rectangle

14. Lateral pressure should be 0.5N for scaling moderate calculus removal. Lateral pressure should be 1-2N for debriding minimal calculus and biofilm.
    a. Both statements are true.
    b. Both statements are false.
    c. The first statement is true, the second statement is false.
    d. The first statement is false, the second statement is true.

15. The point of the ultrasonic tip exerts a concentrated output of force. A true universal ultrasonic tip is not possible.
    a. Both statements are true.
    b. Both statements are false.
    c. The first statement is true, the second statement is false.
    d. The first statement is false, the second statement is true.

16. The operating frequency in kHz of piezoelectric scalers is:
    a. 20
    b. 25
    c. 30
    d. 35

17. All of the following are adaptation patterns used with ultrasonic instrumentation EXCEPT:
    a. Transverse
    b. Horizontal
    c. Oblique
    d. Vertical

CASE STUDY

Your 50-year-old male patient requires periodontal therapy. He presents with moderate calculus supra- and subgingivally. Pocket depths are 4-6 mm generalized with 2-mm recession. Map out your strategy for ultrasonic instrumentation. Include tip types systematic approaches to efficient instrumentation.

_____

_____

_____

_____

_____

_____

_____

_____

_____

_____

_____

_____

_____

_____

30 Root Morphology and Instrumentation Implications

SHORT ANSWER QUESTIONS

1. What is the imaginary vertical line representing the long axis of a tooth in relationship to a horizontal plane?

    a. axial positioning

    _____

    _____

2. What phenomena occurs when there is union of two normally separated tooth germs?

    a. fused roots

    _____

    _____

3. What are extra roots called; often identified through radiographs?

    a. accessory roots

    _____

    _____

4. What are the tiny balls of enamel in the furcation area on maxillary molars and are thought to be due to a genetic error in the developing root sheath as it reaches the furcation area?

    _____

    _____

    _____

5. What is the excessive formation of cementum in the apical third to half of the tooth after the tooth has erupted that may be caused by trauma, chronic inflammation of the pulp, or metabolic disturbances?

    _____

    _____

    _____

FILL IN THE BLANK STATEMENTS

Select the best term from the chapter and complete the following statements.

1. The _____ is part of the dentin covered by cementum and embedded in the alveolar bone, and it begins at the cementoenamel junction.

2. The _____ is the end or tip of the root.

3. The surrounding area of the apex is the _____.

4. The open at the apex whereby nerves and blood vessels enter the pulp canal is the _____.

5. Unbranched portion of multi-rooted teeth is the _____.

6. Branched portion of multi-rooted teeth is a _____.

7. The opening into a furcation is the _____.

8. The most coronal portion of the furcation is the _____.

9. The space between bi- or tri-furcated roots is _____.

10. The _____ is the portion of exposed tooth above the gingival margin.

11. The _____ is the specific anatomical landmark around the perimeter of the tooth where the enamel covering the crown of the tooth meets the cementum covering the root.

MULTIPLE CHOICE QUESTIONS

Complete each question by circling the best answer.

1. Teeth that are egg-shaped with facial surface broader than lingual surface are:
   a. Central incisors
   b. Lateral incisors
   c. Canines
   d. Premolars

2. A sharp bend presents on the root surface of a mandibular left first premolar. This condition is most likely:
   a. Enamel pearl
   b. Hypercementosis
   c. Dilaceration

3. Maxillary first premolars have two roots that are mesially and distally located. Maxillary first premolars have furcations on the mesial and distal sides.
   a. Both statements are true.
   b. Both statements are false.
   c. The first statement is true and the second statement is false.
   d. The first statement is false and the second statement is true.

4. Maxillary molars have all of the following roots EXCEPT:
   a. Palatal
   b. Distolingual
   c. Mesiobuccal
   d. Distobuccal

5. The identification of root anatomy and root surface characteristics during periodontal assessment phase should be identified to plan for care. An understanding of root morphology is necessary for assessment and instrumentation.
   a. Both statements are true.
   b. Both statements are false.
   c. The first statement is true and the second statement is false.
   d. The first statement is false and the second statement is true.

6. The more cervical the furcation is, the more stable the tooth because of root separation. First molar root trunks are shorter than second or third molar root trunks.
   a. Both statements are true.
   b. Both statements are false.
   c. The first statement is true and the second statement is false.
   d. The first statement is false and the second statement is true.

7. Instrument of choice to access a palatogingival groove would be all of the following EXCEPT:
   a. Mini curet
   b. Columbia curet
   c. Micro curet
   d. Extended shank curet

171

8. A cervical enamel projection that extends into the furcation is which CEP grade classification?
   a. I
   b. II
   c. III
   d. IV

9. A universal curet can adapt to all areas of root surfaces. Horizontal location of furcations is the most important aspect of instrument selection.
   a. Both statements are true.
   b. Both statements are false.
   c. The first statement is true and the second statement is false.
   d. The first statement is false and the second statement is true.

31 Dental Implants and Periimplant Care

COMPETENCIES

1. Describe the background of dental implants and discuss the indications, contraindications, and patient selection of dental implants.
2. Explain the basic steps in implant treatment planning, placement, and maintenance.
3. Understand the role of the dental hygienist in relation to implant maintenance.
4. Define peri-implant health, peri-implant mucositis, and peri-implantitis and explain how to make the diagnoses.
5. Detail the need for compliance with proper at-home implant care.
6. Discuss professional maintenance of dental implants.

SHORT ANSWER QUESTIONS

1. The three components of dental implants are:

   _____

   _____

   _____

2. Order the following sequence of the implant timeline:
   Implant is placed in alveolar bone
   Prosthetic fabrication
   Maintenance
   Healing time
   Gingival tissue covers implant surgically
   Incision is made into gingiva/mucosa into underlying bone
   Implant is uncovered and transmucosal abutment is placed

   _____

   _____

   _____

   _____

   _____

   _____

   _____

3. List contraindications for implant placement.

_____

_____

_____

_____

_____

_____

4. List what data is collected about an implant during a maintenance exam.

_____

_____

_____

_____

_____

_____

_____

_____

FILL IN THE BLANK STATEMENTS

Select the best term from the chapter and complete the following statements.

1. _____ is the stable long-term connection of the implant in supportive bone.

2. _____ is space between implant platform and the base of the abutment.

3. _____ is the direct attachment of epithelial and connective tissue to tooth/implant.

4. _____ is reversible inflammation due to biofilm that does not penetrate the supportive bone.

5. _____ is irreversible inflammation resulting in supportive bone degeneration of 2 mm or more.

Complete each question by circling the best answer.

1. All of the following are components of stabilization EXCEPT:
   a. Prosthesis
   b. Bone graft
   c. Implant
   d. Abutment

2. Contraindications to implant placement include all of the following EXCEPT:
   a. Poor homecare
   b. Tobacco use
   c. Diabetes
   d. Bisphosphonate history

3. Virtual treatment planning includes all of the following EXCEPT:
   a. Orthodontics
   b. Site reconstruction
   c. Implant position
   d. Bone density/availability

4. Waiting time for placement of implant after the tooth extraction is:
   a. None
   b. 10 days to 2 weeks
   c. 1-2 months
   d. 3-6 months

5. Waiting time for osseous integration following implant placement is:
   a. None
   b. 10 days to 2 weeks
   c. 1-2 months
   d. 3-6 months

6. All of the following are implant texture macro-geometry EXCEPT:
   a. Threaded
   b. Smooth
   c. Cross hatched
   d. Tapered

7. Stainless steel curettes and scalers are contraindicated for use on implants.
   a. True
   b. False

8. All of the following are elements in diagnosing peri-implant disease EXCEPT:
   a. Suppuration
   b. Bleeding on probing
   c. Probe depths over 3 mm
   d. Clinical attachment level

9. Probing around implants using metal probes is not recommended. Metal probes may scratch the implant and damage epithelial attachment.
   a. Both statements are true.
   b. Both statements are false.
   c. The first statement is true, the second statement is false.
   d. The first statement is false, the second statement is true.

10. The dental hygienist finds 5 mm pocket readings with bleeding and suppuration around an implant replacing tooth number 9. What Human Needs deficit doe this reflect?
    a. Protection from Health Risks
    b. Wholesome Facial Image
    c. Skin and Mucous Membrane Integrity of the Head and Neck
    d. Biologically Sound and Functional Dentition

11. All of the following are true concerning the implant platform EXCEPT:
    a. Internal connection
    b. External connection
    c. Lateral connection
    d. Tissue level
    e. Bone level

12. All of the following are contraindicated for use with titanium implants EXCEPT:
    a. Stainless steel curets
    b. Flour of pumice polishing
    c. Graphite
    d. Ultrasonic scalers

CASE STUDY

Your patient, a 40-year-old female nurse, reports for dental hygiene services. She was seen 2 years ago, when she had an implant replacing tooth #3. This is her first recare visit following implant placement. The patient has moderate biofilm generalized with moderate inflammation. She also has moderate calculus interproximal posterior and mandibular anterior. Probe readings are 4-5 mm posterior with BOP and 3-4 mm anterior. You notice suppuration around the implant with localized 6 mm pockets.

1. What is your dental hygiene diagnosis?
2. What is your dental hygiene treatment plan?
3. What other questions will you ask your patient?
4. What radiographs will you take?
5. What is your education plan?
6. What further action needs to be taken?

_____

_____

_____

_____

_____

_____

_____

_____

_____

_____

_____

_____

32 Tooth Polishing and Whitening

COMPETENCIES

1. Discuss rubber-cup tooth-polishing technique and armamentarium selection for various patient conditions, and perform the procedure on a patient.
2. Discuss air polishing technique and armamentarium options for various patient conditions, and perform the procedure on a patient.
3. Describe client or patient education and motivation in relation to extrinsic stain removal procedures.
4. Discuss teeth whitening including at-home products and in-office techniques. Consider the hygienist's role in in-office whitening procedures.
5. Value the legal and ethical principles that apply to tooth-polishing and whitening services.

SHORT ANSWER QUESTIONS

1. List contraindications for rubber cup polishing.

_____

_____

_____

_____

_____

_____

_____

_____

_____

_____

2. List precautions needed when rubber cup polishing.

_____

_____

_____

_____

_____

_____

_____

_____

_____

_____

177

3. List the contraindications to air polishing.

_____

_____

_____

_____

_____

_____

_____

_____

_____

4. List contraindications to tooth whitening.

_____

_____

_____

_____

_____

_____

_____

_____

_____

_____

_____

_____

_____

_____

_____

_____

5. What is the term for a reaction accompanied by the release of heat?

_____

_____

_____

_____

VIDEO REVIEW QUESTIONS

The following questions are directed toward the tooth polishing and whitening videos located on Evolve. Watch the following videos and answer the questions:

- *Air Polishing Technique*
- *Rubber-Cup Polishing*

1. When is rubber-cup polishing indicated?

_____

_____

2. What type of pressure should be used when performing rubber-cup polishing?

_____

_____

3. What sequence is recommended for rubber-cup polishing?

_____

_____

_____

4. What is the method of action when using the air polisher?

_____

_____

5. What fulcrum is used when holding the air polisher handle?

_____

_____

6. What degree angle is used when directing the air polishing tip – *supragingivally to treat* - prior to posterior teeth?

_____

_____

7. What degree angle is used when directing the air polishing tip – *supragingivally to treat* - prior to anterior teeth?

_____

_____

8. What degree angle is used when directing the air polishing tip to occlusal surfaces of teeth?

_____

_____

FILL IN THE BLANK STATEMENTS

Select the best term from the chapter and complete the following statements.

1. The most appropriate polishing agent for gold foil restorations is _____.

2. A person with heavy brown stain would require _____ as a stain removal.

3. The most effective agent for polishing highly filled hybrid composites is _____.

4. _____ is used to lighten the tooth color of an endodontically treated tooth.

5. _____ removes a thin layer of enamel and uses a paste of abrasives and hydrochloric acid to remove superficial dark stains or decalcified areas of enamel.

6. _____ air polishing powder should be avoided for patients with salt-restricted diets.

MULTIPLE CHOICE QUESTIONS

Complete each question by circling the best answer.

1. Fine prophylaxis paste increases tooth surface sheen. Fine grit is recommended for most patients.
   a. Both statements are true.
   b. Both statement are false.
   c. The first statement is true, the second statement is false.
   d. The first statement is false, the second statement is true.

2. Which procedure is recommended to lighten the color of an endodontically treated tooth?
   a. Coarse grit prophylaxis paste
   b. Intra-coronal bleaching
   c. OTC whitening products
   d. Baking soda and peroxide

3. Which of the following is a contraindication to rubber cup polish?
   a. Severe gingival inflammation
   b. Tobacco stain
   c. Tetracycline stain
   d. Respiratory infection

4. Which of the following is a contraindication to air polish?
   a. Tobacco stain
   b. Coffee stain
   c. Contact lenses
   d. Liver disease

5. Which of the following is a side effect of tooth whitening?
   a. Dissolution of calculus
   b. Decreased pocket depths
   c. Increased biofilm
   d. Sore throat

6. All of the following are contraindications to air polish EXCEPT:
   a. Renal disease
   b. Respiratory disease
   c. Patients requiring pre-med
   d. Patients with a communicable disease

7. All of the following are contraindications to tooth whitening EXCEPT:
   a. Recession
   b. Sensitivity
   c. Caries
   d. Yellow stain

8. All of the following are contraindications to rubber cup polish EXCEPT:
   a. Newly erupted teeth
   b. Dentinal hypersensitivity
   c. Caries
   d. Tea stain

9. Your patient is interested in having whiter teeth. He smokes a pack of cigarettes a day. What Human Needs deficit does this address?
   a. Protection from Health Risks
   b. Freedom from Pain
   c. Wholesome Facial Image
   d. Biologically Sound and Functional Dentition

10. Fine prophylaxis pastes increase tooth surface cleanliness and luster. A fine grit is recommended for coronal polishing for most patients because it facilitates faster stain removal.
    a. Both statements are true.
    b. Both statements are false.
    c. The first statement is true, the second is false.
    d. The first statement is false, the second is true.

11. Which polishing agent is the least abrasive, according to the Mohs Hardness Scale?
    a. Superfine pumice
    b. Calcium carbonate
    c. Tin oxide
    d. Aluminum silicate

At your patient's last appointment 2 weeks ago, she received bleaching trays and 32% carbamide peroxide gel. After using the gel for 2 weeks, she reports that her teeth are extremely sensitive.

1. Will you recommend changing products? If so, what is your alternate recommendation?
2. What is your recommendation for her sensitivity?
3. What other education can you provide for her?

_____

_____

_____

_____

_____

_____

_____

_____

_____

_____

Performance Objective

By following a routine procedure that meets the stated protocols, the student will demonstrate the appropriate technique for **32.1 Rubber Cup Polishing**

Evaluation and Grading Criteria

Instructor will assign grades for each performance criteria.

   <u>3</u> Student competently met stated criteria
   <u>2</u> Student required minimal assistance to meet criteria
   <u>1</u> Student showed uncertainty when attempting criteria
   <u>0</u> Student was not prepared and needs to repeat criteria
<u>N/A</u> Student was not evaluated

Performance Standards

Instructor shall identify steps that are critical with an asterisk (*)

Performance Criteria	*	Self	Peer	Instructor	Comments

Equipment
    Safety glasses for patient
    Personal protective equipment (PPE)
    Polishing paste, aesthetic restoration polishing paste, and
       low-abrasive toothpaste
    Prophylaxis angle and toothbrush
    Low-speed handpiece
    Rubber cups and pointed-bristle brushes
    Mouth mirror, air-water syringe
    Saliva ejector or high-volume evacuation (HVE) tip
    Dental floss or tape
    Floss threader (if needed)
    Gauze squares
    Disclosing solution (optional)					

STEPS *Preparation and Positioning* 1. Evaluate patient's health and pharmacologic history to determine need for precautions or treatment alterations					
2. Identify tooth surfaces indicated and contraindicated for polishing. Always polish aesthetic restorations first, then polish teeth					
3. Educate patient about tooth stains, polishing procedure, and stain prevention (as needed)					
4. Select polishing abrasive based on type of stain and oral restorations and assemble basic setup					
5. Wear appropriate PPE and provide protective eyewear for patient					
6. Have patient tilt head up and turn slightly away when polishing maxillary and mandibular right buccal surfaces of posterior teeth (left buccal if left-handed practitioner) and maxillary and mandibular left lingual surfaces of posterior teeth (right lingual if left-handed practitioner)					

Continued

Performance Criteria	*	Self	Peer	Instructor	Comments
Grasp					
7. Use modified pen grasp					
8. Rest handpiece in V of hand					
9. Have all fingers in contact as a unit					
Fulcrum					
10. Establish fulcrum close to working area					
11. Fulcrum on ring finger					
12. Use moderate fulcrum pressure					
Adaptation					
13. Angle rubber cup to flare at gingival margin and interproximally					
14. Adapt rubber cup to reach distal, facial and lingual, or mesial surfaces					
15. Adapt cup to tooth by rotating handpiece or pivoting on fulcrum as necessary					
16. Adapt brush to occlusal surface					
Stroke					
17. Fill cup with paste and evenly apply to surfaces to be polished					
18. Place cup on tooth; activate handpiece by gently stepping on rheostat. Stroke from the gingival third to the incisal third with just enough pressure to make the cup flare while using wrist-forearm motion to polish the teeth					
19. **Use low speed and intermittent, dabbing, overlapping** strokes with light to moderate pressure in a cervical to occlusal or incisal direction					
20. Remove rubber cup from tooth at completion of stroke; readapt cup for next stroke					
21. Hold mirror in non-dominant hand to retract buccal mucosa. Instruct patient to close mouth halfway and to tilt head slightly toward the ceiling. Polish buccal surfaces of maxillary right posterior quadrant					
22. Polish teeth systematically as indicated. Begin with restorations needing polishing. Then, polish facial surfaces of maxillary teeth, lingual surfaces of maxillary teeth, buccal surfaces of mandibular teeth, and lingual surfaces of mandibular teeth needing coronal polishing					

Performance Criteria	*	Self	Peer	Instructor	Comments
23. Rinse patient's teeth as indicated based on presence of prophylaxis paste					
24. Floss patient's teeth with abrasive agent still on teeth, then rinse					
25. Apply fluoride therapy if indicated					
26. Document completion of service in patient's record under "Services Rendered" and date the entry (e.g., "Removed tobacco stain with rubber-cup polishing on No. 6-11L, 22-27 F and L; patient removed oral biofilm from remaining teeth with a soft toothbrush and fluoride gel toothpaste. Flossed all teeth. Fluoride varnish. Advised patient not to eat, drink, or rinse hot foods or beverages for 4-6 minutes.")					
27. Prevention of Disease Transmission	*				
ADDITIONAL COMMENTS					

Performance Objective

By following a routine procedure that meets the stated protocols, the student will demonstrate the appropriate technique for **32.2 Air Polishing Technique**

Evaluation and Grading Criteria

Instructor will assign grades for each performance criteria.

3 Student competently met stated criteria
2 Student required minimal assistance to meet criteria
1 Student showed uncertainty when attempting criteria
0 Student was not prepared and needs to repeat criteria
N/A Student was not evaluated

Performance Standards

Instructor shall identify steps that are critical with an asterisk (*)

Performance Criteria	*	Self	Peer	Instructor	Comments

Equipment
  Appropriate air-polishing powder and low-abrasive prophy powder
  Appropriate air-polisher device/nozzle and toothbrush
  Dental floss or tape
  Mouth mirror, air-water syringe
  Disclosing solution
  Lubricant for patient's lips
  Saliva ejector and high-volume evacuation (HVE) tip
  Safety glasses for patient
  Personal protective equipment (PPE)					

STEPS *Preparation and Positioning* 1. Evaluate patient's health and pharmacologic history to determine need for antibiotic premedication and contraindications to air polishing					
2. Identify tooth surfaces and restorations indicated and contraindicated for polishing and agents to be used					
3. Identify tooth surfaces and restorations indicated and contraindicated for polishing and agents to be used					
4. Educate patient about air polishing procedure					
5. Assemble high-speed evacuation and saliva ejector					
6. Verify that slurry exits from device tip when held outside the mouth; adjust saliva ejector as necessary					
7. Use appropriate PPE and provide protective eyewear for patient					
8. Clinician, patient, and equipment must be in appropriate position for each area					

Continued

Performance Criteria	*	Self	Peer	Instructor	Comments
Grasp					
9. Use modified pen grasp					
10. Rest handpiece in V of hand					
11. Have all fingers in contact as a unit					
12. Tuck excess cord around pinkie finger, if desired					
Fulcrum					
13. Use external soft-tissue fulcrums					
Adaptation and Stroke for Supragingival with DENTPLSY Cavitron Prophy Jet					
14. Activate foot pedal per manufacturer's instructions for appropriate combined air-water-powder spray					
15. At about 3 to 4 mm from tooth surface and at correct angulation, use constant circular sweeping motions, from proximal to proximal; pivot nozzle to surface being polished; polish several teeth for 1 to 2 seconds each and rinse. Surfaces without stain are cleaned with a toothbrush and low-abrasive toothpaste					
Adaptation and Stroke for Subgingival with Hu-Friedy Air-Flow standard handpiece (1-4 mm)					
16. Activate foot pedal per manufacturer's instructions for appropriate combined air-water-powder spray					
17. At 3 mm from tooth surface and at 45 degree angulation to the gingival margin, use a constant half circle "smiley face" motion, from proximal to proximal moving incisally for 3-5 seconds per tooth. Remove calculus with power and hand scaling					
Adaptation and Stroke for Subgingival with Hu-Friedy Air-Flow with subgingival nozzle (4-9 mm)					
18. Insert tip of nozzle into the depth of the pocket; pull nozzle 1 mm from base					
19. Activate foot pedal per manufacturer's instructions for appropriate combined air-water-powder spray; move nozzle in continuous vertical motion for 5 seconds until nozzle is removed from the pocket. Remove calculus with power and hand scaling					
Other					
20. Rinse with water; floss all teeth (or have patient do so and evaluate their flossing technique)					
21. Evaluate effectiveness with disclosing solution, compressed air, and good lighting					

Performance Criteria	*	Self	Peer	Instructor	Comments
22. Provide professionally applied topical fluoride treatment					
23. Dispose of single-use items according to federal, state, and local regulations					
24. Properly disinfect and sterilize all other equipment					
25. Document completion of service in patient's record under "Services Rendered" and date the entry (e.g., "Removed tobacco stain with supragingival air polishing on No. 6-11L, 22-27L; removed patient oral biofilm from remaining teeth with a soft toothbrush and fluoride toothpaste. Flossed all teeth. APF topical fluoride gel treatment—tray method—provided for 4 minutes. Advised patient not to eat, drink, or rinse for 30 minutes")					
26. Prevention of Disease Transmission	*				
ADDITIONAL COMMENTS					

33 Decision Making Related to Nonsurgical Periodontal Therapy

1. Compare and contrast concepts of dental hygiene care for patients with various classifications of periodontal health and disease, including scaling, oral prophylaxis, root planing, periodontal debridement, host modulation therapy, and therapeutic endpoints.
2. Describe the assessment, diagnosis, and care planning involved with NSPT.
3. Detail the current classifications of periodontal diseases and discuss how each classification might progress and respond to NSPT given risk factors, systemic health, self-care, and adherence to periodontal maintenance recommendations.
4. Discuss oral hygiene instructions for self-care.
5. Describe the process of appointment planning for NSPT and plan implementation of nonsurgical periodontal therapy, including mechanical nonsurgical pocket therapy, chemotherapy for periodontal diseases, and/or full mouth disinfection.
6. List the reasons a patient may need a referral to a periodontist and discuss surgical intervention. Also, discuss the rationale and procedure for reevaluation following NSPT and its relationship to the decision regarding follow-up care including possible referrals.
7. Explain how dental insurance benefit plans relate to case presentations and implementation of nonsurgical periodontal therapy.
8. Consider factors that influence decisions regarding periodontal maintenance therapy and suggest appropriate intervals based on individual patient needs.

SHORT ANSWER QUESTIONS

1. List considerations for frequency of periodontal recare.

_____

_____

_____

_____

_____

2. List eight plaque-retentive factors that contribute to gingivitis and periodontal disease.

_____

_____

_____

_____

_____

3. What are the goals of periodontal therapy?

_____

_____

_____

_____

_____

4. What is the purpose of phase I periodontal therapy?

_____

_____

_____

5. What is host modulation therapy?

_____

_____

_____

6. List the objectives of presenting periodontal therapy cases:

_____

_____

_____

_____

_____

_____

_____

7. The purpose of evaluation and reevaluation after NSPT is:

_____

_____

_____

_____

_____

FILL IN THE BLANK STATEMENTS

Select the best term from the chapter and complete the following statements.

1. A (an) _____ is a preventive procedure that includes supra- and subgingival scaling as well as biofilm and stain removal.

2. _____ is the removal of biofilm, calculus, and retentive factors while preserving as much tooth surface as possible.

3. _____ occurs when there is optimum healing with gingival health, pocket depth reduction, and an improvement in clinical attachment level after nonsurgical periodontal therapy.

4. _____ is a therapeutic procedure to smooth dentin or cementum that contain calculus, toxins, or microorganisms while preserving as much root structure as possible.

5. Periodontal maintenance is also known as _____.

Complete each question by circling the best answer.

1. Stabilizing clinical attachment levels, reducing pocket depths, and restoring gingival health is called:
   a. Host modulation
   b. Therapeutic endpoint
   c. Refractory therapy
   d. Scaling and root planing

2. Gingival and periodontal health is determined by:
   a. Lack of bleeding upon probing
   b. Lack of erythema
   c. Frequency of recare visits
   d. Absence of biofilm

3. Refractory periodontal disease is indicative of which type of treatment?
   a. Prescription fluoride therapy
   b. Bacterial culture with systemic antibiotics
   c. Surgical intervention
   d. Chlorhexidine gluconate delivered via irrigation

4. Most cases of slight to moderate periodontitis can be effectively treated with nonsurgical therapy. Surgery is indicated for all cases of advanced periodontitis.
   a. Both statements are true.
   b. Both statements are false.
   c. The first statement is true, the second statement is false.
   d. The first statement is false, the second statement is true.

5. All of the following additional interventions may be considered when utilizing initial therapy for advanced periodontitis, EXCEPT:
   a. Replacing defective restorations
   b. Removing teeth with poor prognoses
   c. Testing for antibiotic sensitivity
   d. Subgingival microbial analysis

6. When treating aggressive periodontitis:
   a. Surgical intervention is the first course of action
   b. Amount of biofilm and calculus formation determines treatment
   c. Initial nonsurgical therapy alone is most effective
   d. Host response to periodontal pathogens is most important

7. Photodynamic therapy is used to treat aggressive periodontitis. Research has shown no additional benefit when photodynamic therapy is used to treat aggressive periodontitis.
   a. Both statements are true.
   b. Both statements are false.
   c. The first statement is true, the second statement is false.
   d. The first statement is false, the second statement is true.

8. Procedures used in nonsurgical periodontal therapy include all of the following EXCEPT:
   a. Chemotherapy
   b. Radiation therapy
   c. Mechanical nonsurgical pocket therapy
   d. Full mouth disinfection

9. What would be the BEST choice for Human Needs Conceptual model deficit in a patient who presents with generalized moderate periodontal disease, bleeding, pocket depth of 5-6 mm who recently had a knee replacement?
   a. Protection from Health Risks
   b. Skin and Mucous Membrane Integrity of the Head and Neck
   c. Biologically Sound and Functional Dentition
   d. Responsibility for Oral Health

10. All of the following are characteristics of chronic periodontal disease EXCEPT?
    a. Pathogenic bacteria
    b. Initiated by biofilm
    c. Painful
    d. Slow to progress

11. A preventive procedure that uses supra- and subgingival scaling with biofilm and stain removal is:
    a. Oral prophylaxis
    b. Scaling
    c. Periodontal debridement
    d. Scaling and root planing

12. The removal of all subgingival oral biofilm and its by-products, biofilm retentive factors, and calculus-embedded cementum during instrumentation while preserving as much tooth surface as possible is:
    a. Oral prophylaxis
    b. Scaling
    c. Periodontal debridement
    d. Scaling and root planing

13. Gingival health renewal, pocket depth reduction, stable clinical attachment levels after periodontal therapy is:
    a. Periodontal evaluation
    b. Theraputic enpoint
    c. Clinical health
    d. Host modulation

14. The decision to care for a patient in the general dental practice or to refer to a periodontal practice is made on the basis of all the following EXCEPT:
    a. The type, severity, complexity, and grading of the patient's disease
    b. The dental hygienist's experience
    c. The time allotted to maintain periodontally involved cases
    d. The general dentist's experience

CASE STUDY

Your new patient, a 55-year-old male, reports to your office for dental hygiene care. He has not had any professional dental care for over 20 years. He reports that he has not been to a medical doctor in over 10 years. He takes OTC medication for seasonal allergies and acid reflux. He smokes 1 pack of cigarettes a day. Clinical assessment reveals generalized heavy supragingival and subgingival calculus with pocket depths of 4-6 mm generalized with 1-2 mm recession. Generalized moderate bleeding. He reports brushing once a day with a medium toothbrush, and occasionally uses an alcohol-based mouth rinse to freshen his breath. He does not use anything interproximally for plaque removal.

1. What is his periodontal classification?
2. Develop a treatment plan.
3. Explain your education plan for this patient.

_____

_____

_____

_____

_____

_____

_____

_____

_____

_____

_____

_____

34 Acute Gingival and Periodontal Conditions

COMPETENCIES

1. Compare and contrast periodontal and periapical abscesses, including their etiology, signs, symptoms, and treatment.
2. Explain the etiology, signs, symptoms, and treatment of herpetic infections.
3. Discuss the etiology, signs, symptoms, and treatment of pericoronitis.
4. Explain the etiology, signs, and symptoms, and treatment of necrotizing periodontal diseases.

SHORT ANSWER QUESTIONS

1. Describe the change in pathogenic microflora of a periodontal abscess.

_____

_____

_____

_____

2. Describe a gingival abscess.

_____

_____

_____

_____

3. Describe a periodontal abscess.

_____

_____

_____

_____

4. Describe an acute periodontal abscess.

_____

_____

_____

_____

5. Describe a chronic periodontal abscess.

_____

_____

_____

_____

FILL IN THE BLANK STATEMENTS

Select the best term from the chapter and complete the following statements.

1. _____ is the inflammation of the tissue of partially erupted teeth.

2. Diagnostic features of _____ include pain, spontaneous bleeding, necrosis of interdental papillae, and a gray pseudo-membrane.

3. _____ is an accumulation of exudate within a periodontal pocket.

4. A _____ is a long-standing infection that often has opening permitting drainage of the infection.

5. The sinus tract, which is an abnormal channel that connects the abscess to another space or to the surface, is called a _____.

MULTIPLE CHOICE QUESTIONS

Complete each question by circling the best answer.

1. An abscess that is confined to tissue margins in a previously healthy area is:
   a. Gingival
   b. Periodontal
   c. Osseous
   d. Fistulae

2. A periodontal abscess may be associated with all of the following EXCEPT:
   a. Periodontal pocket
   b. Furcation
   c. Operculum
   d. Bone loss

3. A periodontal abscess may be acute or chronic. An acute abscess presents with no symptoms while a chronic abscess presents with pain and swelling.
   a. Both statements are true.
   b. Both statements are false.
   c. The first statement is true, the second statement is false.
   d. The first statement is false, the second statement is true.

4. A chronic periodontal abscess that creates a path connecting infection to another space is:
   a. Pustule
   b. Fistula
   c. Furcation
   d. Pericoronitis

5. Periapical abscess characteristics include all of the following EXCEPT:
   a. Pulpal infection
   b. Pain
   c. Erythema
   d. May follow successful endodontic treatment

6. The MOST important diagnostic tool in determining a periapical abscess is:
   a. Pulp vitality test
   b. Clinical exam
   c. Radiographs
   d. Periodontal probing depths <7 mm

7. Which of the following infections requires a 7-10 day healing time before dental therapy can be provided?
   a. Primary herpetic gingivostomatitis
   b. Periapical abscess
   c. Pericoronitis
   d. Necrotizing ulcerative periodontitis

8. The risks a dental hygienist is exposed to when treating patients with an active oral herpes simplex virus include all of the following EXCEPT:
   a. The dental hygienist is not at risk
   b. Herpetic whitlow
   c. Saliva spatter
   d. Viral transmission on hard surfaces

9. Recurrent herpetic lesions are almost always found on the gingiva or hard palate. Aphthous ulcers are almost always found on moveable mucosa.
   a. Both statements are true.
   b. Both statements are false.
   c. The first statement is true, the second statement is false.
   d. The first statement is false, the second statement is true.

10. A patient reports for routine oral health care. Full mouth radiographs are exposed. A radiolucency is found on the apex of maxillary left incisor. What deficit of the Human Needs Conceptual Model would this reflect?
    a. Protection from Health Risks
    b. Freedom from Pain
    c. Skin and Mucous Membrane Integrity of the Head and Neck
    d. Biologically Sound and Functional Dentition

11. All of the following bacteria are associated with a periodontal abscess EXCEPT:
    a. *Porphyromonas gingivalis*
    b. *Tannerella forsythia*
    c. *Treponema denticola*
    d. *Streptococcus mutans*

12. All of the following are signs and symptoms of a gingival abscess EXCEPT:
    a. Radiographic radiolucency
    b. Erythematous marginal gingival tissue
    c. Pain
    d. Swelling from exudate

CASE STUDY

Your 21-year-old male college student reports to your office complaining of severe intraoral pain and spontaneous gingival bleeding. He reports that he has final exams in a few weeks and is very stressed. Additionally, he has been consuming high amounts of coffee and sugar with very little nutritious meals. His personal hygiene is poor, including lack of routine brushing, and he is sleep-deprived. Your clinical exam reveals severe erythema, cratered papilla, putrid halitosis, thick saliva, and heavy biofilm generalized.

1. What is your dental hygiene diagnosis?
2. Develop a dental hygiene care plan.
3. What other questions could you ask?
4. What is your educational plan for him?
5. What immediate treatment will you perform?

_____

_____

_____

_____

_____

_____

_____

_____

_____

_____

_____

_____

_____

35 Pit and Fissure Sealants

1. Describe the professional development opportunity provided by pit and fissure sealants and the role pit and fissure sealants play in primary and secondary prevention. In addition, discuss retention of sealants and contraindications to sealant placement.
2. Select an appropriate sealant material based on the clinical setting, the oral environment, and the individual needs of the patient.
3. Compare and contrast autopolymerized versus photopolymerized sealants, as well as filled versus unfilled sealants.
4. Describe legal and safety issues related to dental sealants and describe the procedure for sealant placement.

SHORT ANSWER QUESTIONS

1. What sealant material has the most fluoride releasing capability?

_____

_____

_____

2. What sealant material would be best suited for a person with bruxism?

_____

_____

_____

3. What is the average setting time for an auto-polymerized sealant?

_____

_____

_____

4. List the types of acid etch applications.

_____

_____

_____

_____

FILL IN THE BLANK STATEMENTS

Select the best term from the chapter and complete the following statements.

1. The two types of sealants that are hydrophobic are _____ and _____.

2. The two types of sealants that are hydrophilic are _____ and _____.

3. _____ are early carious lesions confined to enamel.

4. _____ are carious lesions that have irreversibly moved into dentin and must be restored.

5. The only type sealant that is hydrophobic is the _____.

MULTIPLE CHOICE QUESTIONS

Complete each question by circling the best answer.

1. Sealants can be auto-polymerizing or photo-polymerizing. Auto-polymerizing sealants have a shorter working time as compared to photo-polymerizing sealants.
   a. Both statements are true.
   b. Both statements are false.
   c. The first statement is true, the second statement is false.
   d. The first statement is false, the second statement is true.

2. Auto-polymerizing sealants are recommended for school-based programs BECAUSE no dedicated equipment is needed.
   a. The first statement is true and the reasoning is true.
   b. The first statement is false and the reasoning is false.
   c. The first statement is false but the reasoning is true.
   d. The first statement is true but the reasoning is false.

3. Which of the following sealant types is self-cured?
   a. Resin based
   b. Resin modifies glass ionomer
   c. Poly-acid modified resin
   d. Glass ionomer cement

4. The most common reason for sealant retention failure is:
   a. Inexpensive sealant material
   b. Salivary contamination
   c. Age of patient
   d. Inexperienced clinician

5. A clinician selects sealant material based on all of the following criteria EXCEPT:
   a. Patient needs
   b. Oral environment
   c. Clinical setting
   d. Amount of visible biofilm in pits/fissures

6. Sharp explorers are recommended for caries detection BECAUSE it is the best way to evaluate the presence of caries.
   a. The first statement is true and the reasoning is true.
   b. The first statement is false and the reasoning is false.
   c. The first statement is false but the reasoning is true.
   d. The first statement is true but the reasoning is false.

7. School-based sealant programs focus on children BECAUSE they typically have newly erupted molars.
   a. The first statement is true and the reasoning is true.
   b. The first statement is false and the reasoning is false.
   c. The first statement is false but the reasoning is true.
   d. The first statement is true but the reasoning is false.

8. A contraindication to sealant placement is:
   a. Childhood asthma
   b. Proximal caries evident on radiographs
   c. Malocclusion
   d. Poor oral hygiene

9. All of the following statements concerning sealants are true EXCEPT:
   a. Act as a physical barrier
   b. Noninvasive
   c. Most commonly applied to newly erupted primary molars
   d. Prevents biofilm from colonizing within pits and fissures

10. Which of the following induces sealants to polymerize?
    a. Free radicals
    b. Acid etch
    c. Bonding agent
    d. Fluoride

11. Sealant placement addresses a deficit in which of the human needs model?
    a. Skin and mucous membrane integrity
    b. Conceptualization and understanding
    c. Biologically sound dentition
    d. Protection from Health Risks

12. What type of sealant is a cement that bond directly to enamel, is hydrophilic, and is used for their fluoride-releasing properties?
    a. Glass ionomer
    b. Resin-based
    c. Polyacid-modified resin
    d. Resin-modified glass ionomer

13. What type of sealant contains particles of glass or quartz to increase the strength and resistance to abrasion and occlusal wear?
    a. Unfilled
    b. Filled
    c. Hydrophobic
    d. Hydrophilic

CASE STUDY

Angelina, a 14-year-old female, presents with generalized heavy biofilm and moderate gingivitis. Pseudo-pockets of 4 mm are present generalized interproximal. Angelina's home has well water. Angelina reports that she brushes once a day and uses nothing for interproximal biofilm removal. She also reports drinking several sodas daily. All first permanent molars have occlusal decay. All second molars are free from decay, but #18 has an operculum.

1. What type of sealant material would be the best choice for Angelina? Why?
2. What specific educational topics would you cover during OHI? Why?

_____

_____

_____

_____

_____

_____

_____

_____

_____

Performance Objective

By following a routine procedure that meets the stated protocols, the student will demonstrate the appropriate technique for applying photo-polymerized sealants.

Evaluation and Grading Criteria

Instructor will assign grades for each performance criteria.

3 Student competently met stated criteria
2 Student required minimal assistance to meet criteria
1 Student showed uncertainty when attempting criteria
0 Student was not prepared and needs to repeat criteria
N/A Student was not evaluated

Performance Standards

Instructor shall identify steps that are critical with an asterisk (*)

Performance Criteria	*	Self	Peer	Instructor	Comments
1. Assembles equipment: a. Mouth mirror b. Explorer c. Cotton forceps d. Traditional or hygoformic saliva ejector e. Sealant kit f. Cotton rolls and rubber dam g. Air-water syringe tip h. Dri-Angles i. High-speed evacuation tube j. Low-speed handpiece or air-polishing device k. Bristled brush l. Pumice m. Floss n. Light protective shield o. Patient protective eyewear p. Personal protective equipment q. Light cure unit r. Round finishing burr s. Articulating paper					
2. Provide patient with filtered protective eyewear. Wear personal protective equipment.					
3. Identify tooth or teeth to be sealed.					
4. Polish the intended surface with a slurry of pumice and water using bristled brush attached to a low-speed handpiece.					
5. Isolate teeth with a rubber dam, or place Dri-Angle over Stensen's duct and insert cotton rolls. Place saliva ejector into patient's mouth.					
6. Dry the site to be sealed with compressed air that is free of oil and moisture.					
7. Apply phosphoric acid to the clean, dry tooth surface. Etch the tooth for 10 to 20 seconds. If using a liquid etch, apply it with a brush. If using a gel etch, apply it and leave undisturbed.					

Continued

Performance Criteria	*	Self	Peer	Instructor	Comments
8. Rinse etched surfaces for 30 to 60 seconds using a water syringe and high-speed evacuation. If gel etch is used, rinse for an additional 30 seconds.					
9. Using cotton forceps, replace cotton rolls and Dri-Angles as they become wet.					
10. Dry the treatment site with compressed air for 10 seconds. Evaluate etched surface.					
11. Apply hydrophilic primer and dry with compressed air.					
12. Apply liquid sealant over the pits and fissures at less than 90 degrees. Allow the sealant to flow into the etched surfaces.					
13. Apply light-cure tip to sealant. Place tip of light source 2 mm from sealant.					
14. Check manufacturer's instructions for time before advancing the light to another area. After the polymerization process, evaluate the sealant with an explorer and check for hard, smooth surface and retention. Set sealant appears as a thin, polymerized film.					
15. Check sealant for imperfections (e.g., incomplete coverage, air bubbles). If detected re-etch tooth for 10 seconds; wash and dry teeth and apply additional sealant material.					
16. Check occlusion with articulating paper to detect high spot areas. Remove excess filled sealant material with a finishing burr.					
17. Remove any residual unsealed liquid sealant with dry gauze. Floss treated teeth.					
18. Apply topical fluoride.					
19. Record type of sealant and teeth sealed in patient's dental record.					
20. Evaluate sealants at each re-care appointment.					
21. Prevention of Disease Transmission.	*				
ADDITIONAL COMMENTS					

36 Nutritional Counseling

COMPETENCIES

1. Apply knowledge about a patient's personal, medical, and dental histories to formulate a comprehensive nutritional assessment.
2. Evaluate a patient's nutritional status using nutritional assessment data and the United States Department of Agriculture's (USDA) MyPlate guidelines.
3. Demonstrate comprehensive and individualized nutritional counseling for individuals at risk of dental caries, periodontal disease, or nutrient deficiencies.
4. Compare and contrast the nutritional needs of various patient populations, including variations in nutritional requirements throughout the life span.

SHORT ANSWER QUESTIONS

1. What is the title of the Dietary Guidelines for Americans by the U.S. Department of Agriculture's (USDA) food guidance system?

_____

_____

2. What specific dietary needs should be increased in the elderly?

_____

_____

_____

_____

3. List the four factors that are needed for dental caries development.

_____

_____

_____

_____

4. How is Body Mass Index calculated?

_____

_____

_____

_____

5. What vitamin deficiency and condition are common in vegans?

_____

_____

_____

_____

6. List reasons why a person would benefit from nutritional counseling

_____

_____

_____

_____

_____

_____

FILL IN THE BLANK STATEMENTS

Select the best term from the chapter and complete the following statements.

1. _____ is comprehensive data collection to identify a patient's need for nutritional counseling and referrals.

2. _____ of a patient's diet may be analyzed by calculating the amount of acid produced in their diet.

3. Elderly patients diagnosed with vitamin B_{12} may develop _____.

4. Weakened collagen formation leading to gingivitis, and poor oral wound healing is an oral sign of a deficiency in _____.

5. Vegetarians should focus on adequate consume adequate amounts of _____.

MULTIPLE CHOICE QUESTIONS

Complete each question by circling the best answer.

1. According to MyPlate, all of the following are used to calculate individual caloric needs EXCEPT:
   a. Activity level
   b. Gender
   c. Age
   d. Race

2. A primary nutritional deficiency is caused by inadequate dietary intake of a nutrient. A secondary nutritional deficiency is caused by a systemic disorder that interferes with the ingestion, absorption, digestion, transport, and use of nutrients.
   a. Both statements are true.
   b. Both statements are false.
   c. The first statement is true, the second statement is false.
   d. The first statement is false, the second statement is true.

3. Artificial sweeteners should be part of the diet of infants or children under age 2. Alternative sweeteners are recommended to infants and children under age 2 because of their anti-cariogenic properties.
   a. Both statements are true.
   b. Both statements are false.
   c. The first statement is true, the second statement is false.
   d. The first statement is false, the second statement is true.

4. The main focus of nutritional counseling for children in the dental setting is:
   a. To screen for obesity
   b. To screen for juvenile diabetes
   c. To assist in caries control
   d. To diagnose a dietary deficiency

5. A dental hygienist may develop a comprehensive meal plan that meets individual dietary patient needs. Quick calculations and charts provided by MyPlate can be used as visual aids for patient education.
   a. Both statements are true.
   b. Both statements are false.
   c. The first statement is true, the second statement is false.
   d. The first statement is false, the second statement is true.

6. An oral sign of deficiency in vitamin B_1 (thiamine) is:
   a. Glossitis
   b. Enamel hypoplasia
   c. Gingival hyperplasia
   d. Cheilitis

7. An oral sign of deficiency in vitamin B_2 (riboflavin) is:
   a. Cheilitis
   b. Candida
   c. Gingivitis
   d. Linea alba

204

Chapter **36** **Nutritional Counseling**

8. An oral sign of deficiency in vitamin B$_{12}$ is:
    a. Edema of pharyngeal and oral mucous membranes
    b. Reduced formation of alveolar bone
    c. Periodontal disease
    d. Disappearance of the filiform and fungiform papillae

9. An oral sign of deficiency in Niacin is:
    a. Defective dentin formation
    b. Smooth shiny tongue
    c. Loss of lamina dura
    d. Caries

10. The BEST Human Needs Conceptual model deficit that addresses a Vitamin C deficiency is:
    a. Biologically Sound and Functional Dentition
    b. Conceptualization and Problem Solving
    c. Responsibility for Oral Health
    d. Skin and Mucous Membrane Integrity of the Head and Neck

11. What vitamin deficiency might present with bleeding, swollen, spongy, erythematous gingival tissue?
    a. A
    b. B
    c. C
    d. D

CASE STUDY

Your patient, a 35-year-old male, presents as a new patient in your office. His health history reveals height of 5'9" and 220 lbs. He reports a family history of diabetes and heart disease. He is taking medication for high blood pressure and anxiety. He states he drinks several sodas a day and has a "sweet tooth."

Comprehensive oral exam reveals:

Generalized severe gingivitis, probe readings of 3-5 mm generalized with bleeding. Clinical and radiographic exam reveals several areas of decay. His tongue appears smooth and shiny.

1. What vitamin deficiencies may he have? Why?
2. Calculate his BMI.
3. How would you collect his dietary history?
4. What online tools would you recommend?
5. When would you refer him to a dietician?
6. Create a comprehensive education plan.

_____
_____
_____
_____
_____
_____
_____
_____
_____
_____
_____

37 Tobacco Cessation

COMPETENCIES

1. Describe the prevalence of the use of tobacco and nicotine products among different segments of the population.
2. Describe adverse systemic and oral health effects of different nicotine and tobacco products in terms as they would be explained to a patient or community group.
3. Accurately communicate to patients the scientific evidence to allow patients to make informed decisions to quit and refrain from using tobacco.
4. Identify various aspects of nicotine addiction.
5. Apply knowledge of treatment programs for nicotine addiction, the Five A's approach, and motivational interviewing for counseling patients to become tobacco-free. In addition, discuss statewide tobacco use quitlines.
6. Evaluate level of dependence and recommend appropriate pharmacologic strategies, including nicotine replacement therapies, to prevent tobacco use and aid in cessation.
7. Encourage local governmental agencies, dental and dental hygiene organizations, community leaders, and insurers to support health promotion and policy making for smoking prevention and cessation, and discuss the dental hygienist's role in the community related to tobacco.

SHORT ANSWER QUESTIONS

1. List the effects of nicotine addiction.

_____

_____

_____

_____

_____

_____

_____

_____

_____

_____

_____

_____

_____

_____

_____

_____

2. What is the 5As approach to assist patients in becoming tobacco-free?

_____

_____

_____

_____

_____

_____

_____

_____

3. What are the OARS tools of change talk?

_____

_____

_____

_____

_____

_____

_____

_____

4. List nicotine replacement therapy examples.

_____

_____

_____

_____

_____

_____

_____

_____

_____

5. List oral tissue changes associated with tobacco use.

_____

_____

_____

_____

_____

_____

6. What are the adverse cardiovascular disease effects of cigarette smoking?

_____

_____

_____

_____

_____

_____

_____

_____

_____

_____

7. What are the adverse effects of cigarette smoking on obstetrics and pediatrics?

_____

_____

_____

_____

_____

_____

_____

_____

_____

8. What are strategies to recommend to patients to cope with cravings and temptation to use tobacco?

_____

_____

_____

_____

_____

_____

_____

_____

_____

_____

_____

_____

_____

FILL IN THE BLANK STATEMENTS

Select the best term from the chapter and complete the following statements.

1. _____ occurs when a person stops tobacco use with the goal of achieving permanent abstinence.

2. _____ is reverting to regular tobacco use after successful tobacco cessation.

3. _____ is a chronic disorder characterized by a vulnerability to relapse that persists for months.

4. _____ is a finely ground tobacco, packaged either loose or in a tea-bag–like sachets.

5. _____ are a nicotine delivery system that converts liquid nicotine into a vapor to stop or cut down on traditional cigarette smoking.

6. _____ provides some blood concentration of nicotine to reduce or eliminate withdrawal symptoms, so clients can focus on the psychosocial and behavioral changes necessary to stop their tobacco use.

7. _____ is form of patient-centered communication to help patients with the ambivalence of an unwanted behavior, so they can start the change process.

8. _____ incorporates the patient's arguments to negative behavioral change.

MULTIPLE CHOICE QUESTIONS

Complete each question by circling the best answer.

1. Free nicotine is deionized nicotine that passes through the oral mucosa into the bloodstream and on to the brain. The higher the pH of a spit tobacco product, the freer nicotine is available.
   a. Both statements are true.
   b. Both statements are false.
   c. The first statement is true and the second statement is false.
   d. The first statement is false and the second statement is true.

2. Nicotine lozenge is contraindicated in all of the following conditions EXCEPT:
   a. Stomach ulcer
   b. Pregnancy
   c. Oral candidiasis
   d. Type I diabetes

3. All of the following are contraindications to the use of the nicotine patch EXCEPT:
   a. Psoriasis
   b. Asthma
   c. Breast feeding
   d. Recent heart attack

4. Smoking harms nearly every organ of the body. Smoking causes several diseases and illnesses.
   a. Both statements are true.
   b. Both statements are false.
   c. The first statement is true and the second statement is false.
   d. The first statement is false and the second statement is true.

5. Tobacco use is the most significant oral risk factor in the development and progression of periodontal disease. Tobacco use is a risk factor for all oral cavity cancers.
   a. Both statements are true.
   b. Both statements are false.
   c. The first statement is true and the second statement is false.
   d. The first statement is false and the second statement is true.

6. Many adults who are diagnosed with depression or anxiety self-medicate with tobacco use. The best treatment for tobacco cessation in patients who have depression or anxiety is nicotine replacement therapy.
   a. Both statements are true.
   b. Both statements are false.
   c. The first statement is true and the second statement is false.
   d. The first statement is false and the second statement is true.

7. Types of nicotine dependence include all the following EXCEPT:
   a. Psychological
   b. Social
   c. Physical
   d. Behavioral

8. Nicotine withdrawal lasts 2-4 months. Pharmacologic interventions can help reduce or eliminate nicotine withdrawal symptoms.
   a. Both statements are true.
   b. Both statements are false.
   c. The first statement is true and the second statement is false.
   d. The first statement is false and the second statement is true.

9. Tobacco addiction is a chronic condition. Repeated cessation treatment in necessary until permanent abstinence is attained.
   a. Both statements are true.
   b. Both statements are false.
   c. The first statement is true and the second statement is false.
   d. The first statement is false and the second statement is true.

10. In-depth tobacco cessation counseling should be offered at every visit. Motivational interviewing is the most effective method in achieving permanent tobacco abstinence.
    a. Both statements are true.
    b. Both statements are false.
    c. The first statement is true and the second statement is false.
    d. The first statement is false and the second statement is true.

11. All the following statements are true about hookah EXCEPT:
    a. Water filters out all the toxins of shisha.
    b. Both tobacco and charcoal smoke are inhaled.
    c. Hookah smokers inhale less smoke than cigarette smokers.
    d. Hookah smokers risk contracting communicable diseases.

12. All the following statements are true about E-cigarettes EXCEPT:
    a. E-cigarettes are not considered a tobacco product.
    b. E-liquids do not contain nicotine.
    c. E-cigarettes are considered less harmful than traditional cigarettes.
    d. FDA classifies E-cigarettes as a tobacco product.

13. All the following are tobacco induced periodontal tissue changes EXCEPT:
    a. Erythematous tissue color
    b. Decreased bleeding
    c. Increased gingival recession around anterior teeth
    d. Increased probing depths

14. All the following are nicotine withdrawal symptoms EXCEPT:
    a. Irritability
    b. Weight loss
    c. Depression
    d. Insomnia

CASE STUDY

Freddy is a 48-year-old healthy Asian male. He reports having his first cigarette at age 12 when he stole a pack from his father. He smoked sporadically throughout high school because he thought he looked "cool." By the time he was 18, he was smoking a pack of cigarettes a day. In college, he admits to smoking 1-2 packs a day and understood that he was addicted but could not stop smoking. He enjoys the feeling of smoking, and it helps him cope with life's stresses. Now he is married and has three children. He realizes that his tobacco use has led to many health problems. He also has periodontal disease and knows it is directly related to smoking. He has tried on many occasions to quit but cannot go more than a week without falling back into his daily routine of smoking.

1. What approach do you take with Freddy? Be specific.
2. How do you help him quit smoking permanently? Develop a plan of action.

38 Impressions for Study Casts and Custom-Made Oral Appliances

COMPETENCIES

1. Define "dental impression," list the main types of dental impressions, and make appropriate clinical judgments regarding the uses of dental impressions in dental hygiene practice, including alginate impressions. Use the criteria for evaluating the acceptability of a dental impression.
2. Discuss dental casts, including gypsum products.
3. Differentiate between the uses and benefits of various custom-made removable oral appliances used by patients for preventive and active dental treatment.
4. Compare and contrast the types of oral surgical splints and stents and their uses.
5. Use patient assessment findings to determine the need for a custom-made oral appliance.
6. Educate patients regarding the maintenance of custom-made oral appliances.

SHORT ANSWER QUESTIONS

1. Briefly explain the procedure of disinfection an impression.

_____

_____

_____

_____

_____

_____

_____

_____

2. List five custom removable oral appliances.

_____

_____

_____

_____

_____

_____

_____

_____

3. List six purposes for patients to wear custom removable oral appliances.

_____

_____

_____

_____

_____

_____

_____

4. Explain the meaning of an irreversible hydrocolloid.

_____

_____

_____

_____

_____

5. Explain the difference between a cast, a diagnostic cast, a working cast, and a die.

_____

_____

_____

_____

_____

_____

6. List the types of athletic mouth guards available.

_____

_____

_____

_____

_____

_____

7. List the negative results of bruxism and clenching.

_____

_____

_____

_____

_____

_____

_____

_____

_____

_____

_____

_____

_____

FILL IN THE BLANK STATEMENTS

Select the best term from the chapter and complete the following statements.

1. _____ is a record of a patient's occlusal relationship usually using wax.

2. A dental hygienist took an alginate impression, left it uncovered, and was unable to pour it up for several hours. The

   resulting distortion of material is called _____.

3. _____ is the uptake of water in the presence of moisture.

4. _____ has very porous crystals that are large and vary in shape. Because of its porosity, it requires the most water when mixing, compared with the other types of gypsum products.

5. _____ is stronger than plaster. Its crystals are uniform in shape, it is smaller and less porous than plaster, and it is used when a stronger working diagnostic cast is needed to make oral appliances, orthodontic retainers and aligners, custom trays, and provisional restorations.

MULTIPLE CHOICE QUESTIONS

Complete each question by circling the best answer.

1. A dental impression is the positive imprint of teeth and surrounding oral structures. A study model is a negative imprint of teeth and oral structures.
   a. Both statements are true.
   b. Both statements are false.
   c. The first statement is true, the second statement is false.
   d. The first statement is false, the second statement is true.

2. The appliance that provides guides for the oral surgeon and the restoring dentist for ideal prosthetic position and angulation of an implant is:
   a. Bite registration
   b. Impression tray
   c. Surgical stent
   d. Mouth guard

3. Alginate material is ideal for final impressions because it provides fine detail.
   a. The statement is true and the reasoning is true.
   b. Both the statement and the reasoning are false.
   c. The statement is true but the reasoning is false.
   d. The statement is false but the reasoning is true.

4. Time needed to mix material, load the tray, and seat the tray in the patient's mouth is called:
   a. Preparation time
   b. Setting time
   c. Imbibition
   d. Working time

5. Diagnostic casts are used to construct oral appliances. Working casts are used for fabrication of prosthetics.
   a. Both statements are true.
   b. Both statements are false.
   c. The first statement is true, the second statement is false.
   d. The first statement is false, the second statement is true.

6. A protective appliance that is designed to withstand recreational impact is:
   a. Athletic guard
   b. Night guard
   c. Day guard
   d. Occlusal guard

7. Decreasing the proportion of water to gypsum stone will result in:
   a. More expansion, less strength
   b. Less expansion, less strength
   c. Less expansion, more strength
   d. More expansion, more strength

8. All of the following are main types of dental impressions EXCEPT:
   a. Preliminary impression
   b. Secondary impression
   c. Final impression
   d. Bite registration

9. Stone casts and plaster models are made of gypsum products. Stone casts are stronger than plaster models.
   a. Both statements are true.
   b. Both statements are false.
   c. The first statement is true, the second statement is false.
   d. The first statement is false, the second statement is true.

10. Your 15-year-old patient reports that he plays soccer on weekends. You recommend an athletic guard. What deficit in the Human Heeds Model does this address?
    a. Protection from Health Risks
    b. Freedom from Fear and Stress
    c. Freedom from Pain
    d. Wholesome Facial Image

Your patient, a 40-year-old female banker, reports that she has a high-stress job and grinds her teeth at night.

1. What other oral manifestations of bruxism might you discover in this patient?
2. What are her treatment options?
3. What educational plan will you present?

_____

_____

_____

_____

_____

_____

_____

_____

_____

_____

_____

Performance Objective

By following a routine procedure that meets the stated protocols, the student will demonstrate the appropriate technique for **Procedure 38-1 SELECTING THE CORRECT TRAY SIZE AND PREPARING IT FOR USE**

Evaluation and Grading Criteria

Instructor will assign grades for each performance criteria.

3 Student competently met stated criteria
2 Student required minimal assistance to meet criteria
1 Student showed uncertainty when attempting criteria
0 Student was not prepared and needs to repeat criteria
N/A Student was not evaluated

Performance Standards

Instructor shall identify steps that are critical with an asterisk (*)

Performance Criteria	*	Self	Peer	Instructor	Comments
EQUIPMENT 　Personal protective equipment 　Antimicrobial mouth rinse 　Lubricating gel 　Maxillary and mandibular impression trays 　Mouth mirror 　Utility wax					
STEPS Preparation 1. Gather all necessary supplies. 2. Position yourself at the side and in front of patient, and seat the patient in an upright position. 3. Explain the procedure to the patient. Have the patient remove any removable oral appliances. 4. Place protective eyewear on the patient. 5. Don personal protective equipment. Disinfect hands and don gloves. 6. Lubricate the patient's lips with a small amount of lubricating gel.					

Continued

Performance Criteria	*	Self	Peer	Instructor	Comments
Mandibular Tray Selection 7. Inspect the patient' mouth to estimate tray size. Note teeth out of alignment, tori/exostosis, and length of dental arch that may require additional tray adaptation for patient comfort. 8. Instruct the patient to tilt chin down. Retract the patient's lip and cheek with index and middle fingers of nondominant hand and at the same time turn the tray sideways and distend the lip and cheek on the opposite side of the mouth with the side of the tray to gain entry into the patient's mouth. Insert the tray with a rotary motion. 9. Assure the tray is centered over the lower teeth by placing the handle at the midline, usually between the central incisors and in line with the center of the chin. 10. Instruct the patient to raise tongue. Lower the tray and at the same time retract the cheek to make certain the buccal mucosa is not caught under the rim of the tray. 11. Check to be sure that the tray covers the teeth and soft tissue. Lift the front of the tray to make certain that the area posterior to the retromolar pad is covered and that there is enough room to allow for 2-3 mm of impression material in the facial and lingual surfaces of the teeth. If necessary, adapt the tray borders with utility (beading) wax to extend into the depth of the vestibule or extend the posterior length of the tray. 12. Reselect larger or smaller tray as needed.					
Maxillary Tray Selection 13. Repeat steps 8 and 9, include an evaluation of the height of the palatal vault. 14. Center the tray by placing the handle between the central incisors in line with the center of the nose. 15. Bring the front of the tray about 2 to 3 mm anterior to the incisors. 16. Seat the tray first by lowering the handle toward the mandibular teeth. 17. Make sure that all the posterior teeth and soft tissue, including the maxillary tuberosity, are covered. Check that laterally there is enough room to allow for a 2 to 3 mm space between the inside of the tray and the facial and lingual surfaces of the teeth. 18. Retract the patient's lip and raise the anterior portion of the tray into place. The tray should fit to the depth of the vestibule and not impinge on soft tissue. 19. Reselect larger or smaller tray as needed.					
Prevention of Disease Transmission	*				
ADDITIONAL COMMENTS					

Performance Objective

By following a routine procedure that meets the stated protocols, the student will demonstrate the appropriate technique for **38-2 mixing alginate.**

Evaluation and Grading Criteria

Instructor will assign grades for each performance criteria.

  3 Student competently met stated criteria
  2 Student required minimal assistance to meet criteria
  1 Student showed uncertainty when attempting criteria
  0 Student was not prepared and needs to repeat criteria
N/A Student was not evaluated

Performance Standards

Instructor shall identify steps that are critical with an asterisk (*)

Performance Criteria	*	Self	Peer	Instructor	Comments

EQUIPMENT
  Personal protective equipment
  Alginate powder
  Measuring scoop
  Room temperature water
  Vial for measuring water
  Wide-blade mixing spatula
  Rubber mixing bowl					

1. Read the manufacturer's directions for the dispensing and manipulation of the alginate.					
2. Place one measure of room-temperature water into the mixing bowl for each scoop of alginate. Check temperature of water to assure it is room temperature. Use warmer warmer water to accelerate the mix and cooler water to slow the setting of the mix.					
3. Shake or fluff the alginate by tipping the container two or three times.					
4. Overfill the correct scoop with powder; tap the scoop with the side of the spatula. Scrape the excess from the scoop with the spatula.					
5. Sift the powder into the water, and stir this with the spatula until all the powder is moist.					
6. Cup the rubber bowl in the palm of your hand with the opening of the bowl facing your wrist. Firmly spread the alginate between the spatula and the side of the rubber bowl. Spatulate the mixture vigorously using a back-and-forth hand motion, spreading the material against the sides of the bowl. Use both sides of the spatula, and rotate the bowl with your fingers during spatulation.					

Continued

219

Performance Criteria	*	Self	Peer	Instructor	Comments
7. Spatulate vigorously for 30 seconds for fast-set products and gather the material together. Use the spatula to crush the mixture and spread it out again. Repeat until a smooth, creamy consistency is achieved within the designated mixing time for either the normal-set or fast-set alginate.					
8. Gather the material into one mass, and wipe it on the inside edge of the mixing bowl.					
9. Prevention of Disease Transmission	*				
ADDITIONAL COMMENTS					

Performance Objective

By following a routine procedure that meets the stated protocols, the student will demonstrate the appropriate technique for **38-3 making a mandibular preliminary impression.**

Evaluation and Grading Criteria

Instructor will assign grades for each performance criteria.

<u>3</u> Student competently met stated criteria
<u>2</u> Student required minimal assistance to meet criteria
<u>1</u> Student showed uncertainty when attempting criteria
<u>0</u> Student was not prepared and needs to repeat criteria
<u>N/A</u> Student was not evaluated

Performance Standards

Instructor shall identify steps that are critical with an asterisk (*)

Performance Criteria	*	Self	Peer	Instructor	Comments

EQUIPMENT
  Personal protective equipment
  Antimicrobial rinse
  Occupational Safety and Health Administration (OSHA)–approved disinfectant
  Alginate powder
  Measuring scoop
  Water Dispenser
  Wide-blade mixing spatula
  Rubber mixing bowl
  Selected and adapted mandibular impression tray
  Saliva ejector					

PREPARATION					
1. Gather all necessary supplies. Seat the patient upright and explain the procedure. Have patient remove any removable oral appliances.					
2. Check the patient's health history to determine any risk factor that may complicate the procedure.					
3. Place protective eyewear on the patient.					
4. Don personal protective equipment.					
5. Lubricate the patient's lips with a small amount of moisturizer.					
6. Combine two measures of room-temperature water with two scoops of alginate, and mix the alginate.					
LOADING THE TRAY					
7. Quickly gather half the alginate in the bowl onto the spatula. Wipe the alginate onto one side of the tray from the lingual side, working from the posterior toward the anterior. Fill to an area just below the rim. Quickly press the material down to the base of the tray.					

Continued

Performance Criteria	*	Self	Peer	Instructor	Comments
8. Gather the remaining half of the alginate in the bowl onto the spatula and load the other side of the tray in the same way.					
9. Moisten your fingers with cold water and smooth over alginate. Make a slight indentation where teeth will insert.					
10. Ask the patient to suck in the saliva in their mouth and swallow.					
11. Take a small amount of impression mixture from the spatula and quickly apply to the occlusal surfaces of the teeth, undercut areas, and vestibular areas.					
SEATING THE TRAY					
12. Place yourself at the 8-o'clock position (4-o'clock position if left-handed), and ask the patient to tilt his or her chin down making the occlusal plane parallel to the floor.					
13. Turn the impression tray sideways.					
14. Retract the patient's lip and cheek with fingers of nondominant hand. Turn the tray sideways when placing it in the mouth, and distend the lip and cheek on the opposite side of the mouth with the side of the tray.					
15. Center the tray over the teeth, and center the handle in line with the center of the patient's chin.					
16. Align the tray 2 to 3 mm anterior to the incisors. Press down the posterior portion of the tray first and then seat the anterior portion of the tray directly down. Instruct the patient to raise their tongue.					
17. Instruct the patient to relax his or her lips and to breathe normally.					
18. Hold the tray steady in place until the material has gelled. Apply firm bilateral pressure with the middle fingers, and use the thumbs to support the jaw.					
REMOVING THE IMPRESSION					
19. Place the fingers of nondominant hand on top of the tray. The index finger of the nondominant hand rests on the incisal surface of the maxillary anterior teeth.					
20. Move the index finger of other hand along the buccal mucosa posteriorly between the impression and the peripheral tissues. The index finger is placed under the posterior facial portion of the tray to lift the tray and break the seal between the impression and the teeth. Grasp the handle of the tray with the thumb and index finger of the dominant hand, and use a firm lifting motion.					

222

Chapter **38** **Impressions for Study Casts and Custom-Made Oral Appliances**

Performance Criteria	*	Self	Peer	Instructor	Comments
21. Remove the tray by turning it slightly sideways to remove it from the patient's mouth.					
22. Evaluate the impression for accuracy.					
POST-IMPRESSION CARE					
23. Give the patient water to rinse their mouth.					
24. Gently rinse debris from the impression under a stream of cold water.					
25. Spray the impression with an approved disinfectant within 10 to 15 minutes. Follow the manufacturer's recommended procedure.					
26. Wrap the impression in a moist paper towel and place it in a precaution bag before pouring it up or in a humidor; label with patient's name. Prepare the laboratory prescription if sending the impressions to the dental laboratory.					
27. Remove any remaining alginate from patient's mouth with floss, scaler, or explorer.					
28. Remove any alginate from patient's face and lips with a warm cloth.					
29. Return any removable oral appliances to patient.					
30. Document completion of this service in the patient's electronic record under "Services Rendered."					
Prevention of Disease Transmission	*				
ADDITIONAL COMMENTS					

COMPETENCY CHAPTER 38 IMPRESSIONS FOR STUDY CASTS AND CUSTOM APPLIANCES

Performance Objective

By following a routine procedure that meets the stated protocols, the student will demonstrate the appropriate technique for **38-4 making a maxillary preliminary impression.**

Evaluation and Grading Criteria

Instructor will assign grades for each performance criteria.

3 Student competently met stated criteria
2 Student required minimal assistance to meet criteria
1 Student showed uncertainty when attempting criteria
0 Student was not prepared and needs to repeat criteria
N/A Student was not evaluated

Performance Standards

Instructor shall identify steps that are critical with an asterisk (*)

Performance Criteria	*	Self	Peer	Instructor	Comments
EQUIPMENT Personal protective equipment Antimicrobial rinse Occupational Safety and Health Administration (OSHA)–approved disinfectant Alginate powder Measuring scoop Water Dispenser Wide-blade mixing spatula Rubber mixing bowl Selected and adapted maxillary impression tray Saliva ejector					
PREPARATION					
1. Gather all necessary supplies. Seat and prepare the patient.					
2. Measure three units of room-temperature water and three scoops of alginate, and mix the alginate.					
LOADING THE TRAY					
3. Load the maxillary tray in one large increment. Load from the posterior end of tray. Use a wiping motion to bring the material forward with the spatula, being careful to place the bulk of the material in the anterior palatal area of the tray. Fill to an area just below the edge of the wax rim.					
4. Be careful not to overfill the posterior portion of the tray that rests against the palate.					
5. Moisten your fingers with water, and smooth surface of the alginate.					
SEATING THE TRAY					
6. Position yourself at the 11-o'clock position (1-o'clock position if left-handed), and instruct the patient to tilt head forward and chin down making occlusal plane parallel to the floor.					

Continued

225

Copyright © 2025 by Elsevier Inc. All rights are reserved, including those for text and data mining, AI training, and similar technologies.

Chapter **38** Impressions for Study Casts and Custom-Made Oral Appliances

Performance Criteria	*	Self	Peer	Instructor	Comments
7. Retract the lips and cheek with fingers of nondominant hand. With the dominant hand, turn the impression tray sideways and at the same time distend the lip and cheek on the opposite side of the mouth with the side of the tray.					
8. Center the tray over the patient's teeth, and center the handle at the midline in line with the center of the patient's nose.					
9. Seat the back of the tray against the posterior border of the hard palate to form a seal. Place the tray ¼ inch or 6 mm anterior to incisors, and seat posterior to anterior direction with a slight vibratory motion.					
10. Gently move the patient's lips up and over the tray as it is seated.					
11. Place your middle fingers over the premolar areas, and hold the lip out with the index finger and the thumb.					
12. Instruct the patient to breathe slowly through the nose and to form an "O" with his or her lips.					
13. Hold the tray in place until the material has completely gelled.					
REMOVING THE IMPRESSION					
14. Place an index finger under the posterior facial portion of the tray to break the seal between the impression and the teeth.					
15. Place the index finger of the nondominant hand on the incisal surface of the mandibular anterior teeth.					
16. Move index finger of other hand along the buccal mucosa posteriorly between the impression and the peripheral tissues. The index finger is placed under the rim of the tray to lift and break the seal between the impression and the teeth. Grasp the handle of the tray with the thumb and index finger of the dominant hand to lower it from the maxillary teeth.					
17. Remove the tray by turning it sideways to take it out of the patient's mouth.					
18. Evaluate the impression for accuracy.					
POST-IMPRESSION CARE					
19. Give the patient water to rinse their mouth.					
20. Gently rinse debris from the impression under a stream of cold water.					

Performance Criteria	*	Self	Peer	Instructor	Comments
21. Spray the impression with an approved disinfectant within 10 to 15 minutes. Follow the manufacturer's recommended procedure.					
22. Wrap the impression in a moist paper towel and place it in a precaution bag before pouring it up or in a humidor; label with patient's name. Prepare the laboratory prescription if sending the impressions to the dental laboratory.					
23. Remove any remaining alginate from patient's mouth with floss, scaler, or explorer.					
24. Remove any alginate from patient's face and lips with a warm cloth.					
25. Return any removable oral appliances to patient.					
26. Document completion of this service in the patient's electronic record under "Services Rendered."					
Prevention of Disease Transmission	*				
ADDITIONAL COMMENTS					

Performance Objective

By following a routine procedure that meets the stated protocols, the student will demonstrate the appropriate technique for **38-5 making a wax bite registration.**

Evaluation and Grading Criteria

Instructor will assign grades for each performance criteria.

<u>3</u> Student competently met stated criteria
<u>2</u> Student required minimal assistance to meet criteria
<u>1</u> Student showed uncertainty when attempting criteria
<u>0</u> Student was not prepared and needs to repeat criteria
<u>N/A</u> Student was not evaluated

Performance Standards

Instructor shall identify steps that are critical with an asterisk (*)

Performance Criteria	*	Self	Peer	Instructor	Comments

EQUIPMENT
  Personal protective equipment
  Bite registration wax (baseplate wax or wax wafer)
  Wide-blade laboratory knife
  Heat source (warm water, Bunsen burner, or torch)
  Occupational Safety and Health Administration (OSHA)–
  approved disinfectant					

PREPARATION					
1. Gather all necessary supplies. Seat the patient upright and explain the procedure.					
2. Reassure the patient that the wax will be warm, not hot.					
3. Measure the length of the wax needed by placing the wax over the biting surfaces of the teeth. If the wax extends past the last tooth, use the laboratory knife to shorten its length after removing the wax from the patient's mouth.					
4. Soften the bite registration wax in hot water or with another heat source (e.g., Bunsen burner or torch).					
SEATING					
5. Place the softened warm wax over the maxillary occlusal surfaces and instruct the patient to bite together on posterior teeth gently and naturally into the wax.					
6. Allow the wax bite to cool in the mouth. If necessary, air from the air-water syringe can be used to cool the wax.					
REMOVAL					
7. Remove the wax carefully when it has cooled.					

Continued

Performance Criteria	*	Self	Peer	Instructor	Comments
POST-WAX BITE CARE					
8. Inspect the wax to be sure it represents the patient's bite. Chill in cold water until firm.					
9. Write the patient's name on a piece of paper and keep it with the wax-bite registration.					
10. Disinfect wax-bite registration with an OSHA-approved disinfectant.					
11. Store the wax-bite registration with the impressions or casts until it is needed for the trimming of the casts.					
12. Document completion of this service in the patient's electronic record under "Services Rendered."					
Prevention of Disease Transmission	*				
ADDITIONAL COMMENTS					

Performance Objective

By following a routine procedure that meets the stated protocols, the student will demonstrate the appropriate technique for **38-6 constructing a custom-made oral appliance for a single-layer mouth guard, Fluoride tray, or tooth-whitening tray.**

Evaluation and Grading Criteria

Instructor will assign grades for each performance criteria.

3 Student competently met stated criteria
2 Student required minimal assistance to meet criteria
1 Student showed uncertainty when attempting criteria
0 Student was not prepared and needs to repeat criteria
N/A Student was not evaluated

Performance Standards

Instructor shall identify steps that are critical with an asterisk (*)

Performance Criteria	*	Self	Peer	Instructor	Comments
Gather Armamentarium a. Personal protective equipment b. Petrolatum lubricant, silicone lubricant c. Polyurethane d. Mouth guard 4 × 4 square e. Long-shank acrylic burr in a laboratory engine f. Matches g. Diagnostic casts h. Crown and collar scissors i. Hanau torch j. Vacuum forming machine k. Laboratory knife					
1. Don personal protective equipment.					
2. Trim the diagnostic cast so that the base extends 3 to 4 mm past the gingival border and the vertical height is minimal. Spray the cast with silicone lubricant.					
3. Place the vacuum forming machine under a hood fan for control of organic emissions.					
4. Prepare the machine. The perforated vacuum plate and the sides of the hinged frame must be lightly sprayed with silicone lubricant.					
5. Open the hinged frame, and center the polyurethane material onto the lower frame.					
6. Close the frame and secure the frame with the latch knob.					
7. Grasp both handles of the locked, hinged frame and lift it until it clicks into position approximately 3 inches above the vacuum plate.					
8. Swing the heating unit to the center position and turn on the heating element switch at the base of the unit.					

Continued

231

Performance Criteria	*	Self	Peer	Instructor	Comments
9. Center cast on the vacuum plate. Some units have extra holes at the front and back of the machine; place the cast between these holes.					
10. Do not leave the machine unattended. Watch the material as it heats for 1 to 2 minutes until it sags ½ inch below the hinged frame.					
11. Grasp both handles of the hinged frame and pull it down over the vacuum plate. The material will be draped over the cast.					
12. Turn on the vacuum motor for 10 seconds.					
13. Swing the heating unit out of the way and turn off the switch.					
14. Turn off the vacuum switch. Release the hinged frame knob and open the frame and hold by the edges to remove it from the vacuum plate.					
15. Hold the splint and cast under running, cold water for at least 30 seconds.					
16. Cut excess material just below the depth of the periphery to remove it from the cast.					
17. Use small, sharp crown and collar scissors to trim approximately 0.5 mm away from the gingival margin.					
18. Place the mouth guard back on the cast.					
19. If necessary, place a thin coat of petroleum jelly on the facial surfaces. Use a low flame to gently readapt the margins so that they cover the entire tooth, but do not overlap the gingivae.					
20. Wearing a mask and safety goggles, trim the mouth guard with an acrylic burr in a laboratory engine.					
21. Polish the edge until smooth with an abrasive and cloth wheel on a lathe or handpiece.					
Prevention of Disease Transmission	*				
ADDITIONAL COMMENTS					

39 Restorative Therapy

COMPETENCIES

1. Discuss the variety of educational requirements that can provide pathways for licensure for dental hygienists and other dental personnel to practice restorative dentistry. In addition, describe the collaborative role of the dental hygienist in restorative dentistry.
2. Detail the rationale for restorative therapy.
3. Describe both direct and indirect restorations, and list the principles of cavity classification and preparation.
4. Discuss the rationale, moisture control, accessibility, visibility, disadvantages, and contraindications of dental isolation.
5. Apply knowledge of why the type of restorative material, location of restoration, and presence of a proximal contact aid in appropriate decisions regarding a matrix system.
6. Describe bonding agents, bases, liners, and cavity sealers.
7. Compare and contrast the differences between amalgam and composite materials and techniques including: preparation design, matrix systems, armamentarium differences, and finishing techniques.
8. Describe intermediary crowns, gingival retractions, temporary or interim restorations, and luting agents.
9. Discuss why the restorative care cycle demands ongoing assessment, evaluation, documentation, and continued care.

SHORT ANSWER QUESTIONS

1. Define indirect restoration and give an example.

_____

_____

_____

_____

2. List three types of materials used for restorative treatment.

_____

_____

_____

_____

3. What type of clinician may provide restorative treatment (in some states) after the dentist treatment plans and prepares the tooth for a restoration?

_____

_____

4. What type of clinician provides more expanded dental care that includes cavity preparations, removal of decay, placement of direct restorations, and simple extractions, under the supervision of a consulting dentist?

_____

_____

_____

_____

5. List five contraindications to using dental dam.

_____

_____

_____

_____

FILL IN THE BLANK STATEMENTS

Select the best term from the chapter and complete the following statements.

1. A defective restoration caused by improper placement by the clinician is considered _____.

2. _____ is placed in the deepest areas of the cavity preparation to provide protection for the pulp and to provide support beneath restorations.

3. _____ are used to seal dentinal tubules and to protect the pulp from chemical irritation.

4. _____ resists tarnish and corrosion.

5. Using _____ relaxes the gingival tissue and the gingival sulcus, allowing impression material into the gingival spaces to capture the gingival margins of the indirect restoration preparation.

MULTIPLE CHOICE QUESTIONS

Complete each question by circling the best answer.

1. Restorative therapy providers include all of the following EXCEPT:
   a. RFE
   b. CDA
   c. DHT
   d. EFDA

2. Restorative therapy includes all of the following EXCEPT:
   a. Occlusal adjustments
   b. Replacing defective restorations
   c. Making esthetic changes
   d. Adjusting tooth morphology

3. Posterior composite restorations are placed instead of amalgam restorations because:
   a. Composites are easier to place
   b. Amalgams have a shorter life span
   c. Composites have fewer incidences of recurrent caries
   d. Patients prefer esthetics of composites

4. All of the following are considerations in matrix system choice EXCEPT:
   a. Proximal contact
   b. Type of restoration to be used
   c. Dental dam clamp interference
   d. Occlusion

5. All of the following are components of current amalgam restorations EXCEPT:
   a. Copper
   b. Tin
   c. Zinc
   d. Lead

6. All of the following are true concerning the smear layer EXCEPT:
   a. Tooth particles left following the cavity preparation
   b. Has no effect on dentin bond strength
   c. May be removed by acid etch
   d. Occurs when dentin is prepped

7. A matrix is needed for all of the following restoration classifications EXCEPT:
   a. II
   b. III
   c. IV
   d. V

8. Bases and liners aid in:
   a. Releasing fluoride over time
   b. Insulation under restoration
   c. Adding bonding strength to restoration
   d. Prevent recurrent decay

9. Which statement is correct concerning composites bonding to tooth structure?
   a. Bonding agents are hydrophobic
   b. Only required with anterior teeth
   c. Not always necessary
   d. Enamel bonding is more predictable than dentin bonding

10. Your patient presents with maxillary anterior teeth that have multiple composite restorations. She is concerned that the color of the restorations has become dark over time and would like to discuss crowns. What deficit of the Human Needs Model does this address?
    a. Freedom from Fear and Stress
    b. Freedom from Pain
    c. Wholesome Facial Image
    d. Skin and Mucous Membrane Integrity of the Head and Neck

11. All of the following may interfere with placement of a composite restoration EXCEPT:
    a. Saliva
    b. Blood
    c. Water
    d. Preprocedural rinse

12. Which of the following is an indirect restoration?
    a. CAD CAM zirconium crown
    b. Anterior composite
    c. Posterior composite
    d. Occlusal amalgam

CASE STUDY

Your 62-year-old patient reports for her 6-month recare appointment. Health history indicates chronic asthma and moderate to severe arthritis in her hands. She states she has difficulty brushing and flossing. Oral exam revealed moderate generalized biofilm and slight calculus localized to mandibular anterior teeth. Several areas of demineralization are apparent on posterior line angles. Probe readings are 3 mm or less. Radiographs reveal MO decay on tooth #4 and DO decay on tooth #19.

1. What restorative material would you choose for this patient? Why?
2. What matrix system would you choose? Why?
3. Would using a dental dam be indicated?
4. What oral hygiene education would you provide? Why?

Performance Objective

By following a routine procedure that meets the stated protocols, the student will demonstrate the appropriate technique for **Procedure 39.1 Placing a Tofflemire Matrix System and Wedge**

Evaluation and Grading Criteria

Instructor will assign grades for each performance criteria.

3 Student competently met stated criteria
2 Student required minimal assistance to meet criteria
1 Student showed uncertainty when attempting criteria
0 Student was not prepared and needs to repeat criteria
N/A Student was not evaluated

Performance Standards

Instructor shall identify steps that are critical with an asterisk (*)

Performance Criteria	*	Self	Peer	Instructor	Comments
EQUIPMENT Personal protective equipment Protective eyewear for client Tofflemire retainer Matrix bands Wooden wedges Metal-cutting scissors Cotton forceps Modeling compound Burnishing instrument Tofflemire matrix system					
STEPS 1. Evaluate the prepared tooth.					
2. Select a matrix band that best encloses all lateral aspects of the cavity and extends 1 to 2 mm above the adjacent marginal ridge and 1 mm beyond the gingival margin.					
3. Select a matrix retainer.					
4. Loop band in fingers so that ends match. The convergent opening (smaller) of the loop should be positioned next to the gingiva (rubber dam).					
5. Position locking vise approximately ¼ inch from end of retainer and free locking screw (spindle) from band slot in the locking vise.					
6. Position loop in retainer (leading with the occlusal edge of the band); insert matched ends into the slots in the locking vise and the loop into the appropriate guide channel. When positioned, the guide channels of the retainer open toward the gingiva. The loop of band should exit guide channel to allow the loop to be positioned from the preferred side of the tooth (usually the facial side).					

Continued

Performance Criteria	*	Self	Peer	Instructor	Comments
7. When inserting band into the retainer, first insert the wider occlusal aspect of the band so that the retainer is seated with the slots of the retainer toward the gingiva.					
8. Shape matrix loop into a rounded form: (1) insert an instrument handle through the loop, (2) pinch the band between the instrument handle and your thumb, and (3) rotate your wrist as you pinch the band.					
9. Position loop around tooth with slots of the Tofflemire and narrow aspect of band toward the gingiva; brace lingual aspect of loop with thumb of opposite hand; gently tighten band by rotating the adjusting nut (larger nut).					
10. Examine placement of band to ensure that band extends occlusally 1 to 2 mm beyond the adjacent marginal ridge; it also should extend apically approximately 1 mm beyond the gingival margin without impinging on soft tissue.					
11. Moisten wedge(s) and place into the lingual embrasure between band and adjacent tooth, slightly beyond the gingival margin. Apply steady pressure on base of the wedge to move it in a facial direction to desired position. Numerous pretrimmed wedges are available for selection.					
12. Burnish internal aspect of band against the adjacent tooth (or teeth) with a thin, rigid instrument.					
13. Conduct a final evaluation of cavity preparation with matrix system in place.					
14. Prevention of Disease Transmission	*				
ADDITIONAL COMMENTS					

Performance Objective

By following a routine procedure that meets the stated protocols, the student will demonstrate the appropriate technique for **Procedure 39.2 Placing an Amalgam Restoration**

Evaluation and Grading Criteria

Instructor will assign grades for each performance criteria.

<u>3</u> Student competently met stated criteria
<u>2</u> Student required minimal assistance to meet criteria
<u>1</u> Student showed uncertainty when attempting criteria
<u>0</u> Student was not prepared and needs to repeat criteria
<u>N/A</u> Student was not evaluated

Performance Standards

Instructor shall identify steps that are critical with an asterisk (*)

Performance Criteria	*	Self	Peer	Instructor	Comments
EQUIPMENT 　Personal protective equipment 　Protective eyewear for client 　Isolation materials 　Triturator 　Amalgam well 　Amalgam carrier 　Amalgam capsules 　Condensing instruments 　Tofflemire matrix system 　Carving and burnishing instruments 　Articulating paper					
STEPS 15. Pretest access to cavity by holding condenser nibs in confined areas of preparation to verify accurate condenser selection.					
16. Adjust triturator settings for speed and time of mix, according to manufacturer's recommendations.					
17. Secure amalgam capsule in triturator locking device; close protective lid.					
18. Mix amalgam, then remove capsule; open it over a catch tray and dispense mix into the amalgam well.					
19. Examine mixed amalgam; note time, or set a timer for 3 minutes.					
20. Load small end of amalgam carrier; dispense a portion into the most confined area of the preparation.					
21. Using small condensers and a stable hand position, firmly adapt the amalgam into all internal cavity features and over margins.					

Continued

239

Performance Criteria	*	Self	Peer	Instructor	Comments
22. Continue to add increments; gradually increase condenser size; remove any "mercury-rich" surface by lateral scooping motions of the condenser nib.					
23. Triturate fresh amalgam as needed; continue to add increments and condense, to build a moderate excess over cavity margins.					
24. Rub and grossly shape the occlusal surface with a few firm strokes using a large ball or egg-shaped burnisher.					
25. Carve and suction away excess amalgam.					
26. Establish marginal ridge height and outer contours next to matrix band by carving with an explorer or similar fine, sharp instrument. Carve excess amalgam away rapidly and recover occlusal margins.					
27. Release matrix band from retainer by loosening band tightener and locking nut; remove wedges.					
28. While maintaining gentle pressure on marginal ridge with a large amalgam condenser, lift matrix band from unrestored proximal area first, then finally from the restored area.					
29. Explore gingival margin for excess (overhang); carve away excess with a fine-bladed instrument (an interproximal carver).					
30. Carve proximal and outer contours to final form. Recover all margins. At margins, all cutting strokes should be directed parallel to margins to maintain a seal and avoid overcarving. Tooth surface is used as a guide by resting the carving edge on it as shaving strokes are made. Carve occlusal anatomy to general form, keeping pits and grooves shallow.					
31. Remove rubber dam; caution client against biting at this time.					
32. Wipe client's lips; suction mouth to remove saliva; isolate operating site with cotton rolls.					
33. Insert articulating paper over area and have client "gently tap back teeth together."					
34. Carve away marking spots on the amalgam until centric occlusion is reestablished as it was before the procedure; re-mark the occlusion as necessary, carving away high spots each time with a carver or round bur, if the amalgam has set up.					

Performance Criteria	*	Self	Peer	Instructor	Comments
35. Insert ribbon and have client gently grind the back teeth; make sure the client moves teeth in all functional directions. Remove markings until presurgical contacts are restored.					
36. Finalize carving and burnish carved amalgam to create smooth finish. Rinse and suction away all debris; caution client to avoid chewing on restored tooth for 24 hours.					
37. After putting client in an upright position, have client "tap-tap-tap" again, then look at the new restoration for shiny spots. Repeat procedure; have client grind the teeth for lateral movement. Adjust high spots as necessary.					
38. Caution client that discernable high spots should be adjusted to avoid fracture.					
39. Prevention of Disease Transmission	*				
ADDITIONAL COMMENTS					

Performance Objective

By following a routine procedure that meets the stated protocols, the student will demonstrate the appropriate technique for **Procedure 39.3 Placing and Finishing a Class II Composite**

Evaluation and Grading Criteria

Instructor will assign grades for each performance criteria.

3 Student competently met stated criteria
2 Student required minimal assistance to meet criteria
1 Student showed uncertainty when attempting criteria
0 Student was not prepared and needs to repeat criteria
N/A Student was not evaluated

Performance Standards

Instructor shall identify steps that are critical with an asterisk (*)

Performance Criteria	*	Self	Peer	Instructor	Comments

EQUIPMENT
  Personal protective equipment
  Protective eyewear for patient
  Isolation materials
  Glass ionomer cavity liner or sealer as needed
  Conditioning agent (acid gel)
  Priming agent
  Bonding resin
  Composite
  Resin surface coating
  Matrix system-Sectional matrix system or Tofflemire retainer
    with precontoured band
  Dispensing syringe
  Curing light and protective shields
  Plastic instruments
  Finishing burs and discs
  Articulating paper					

STEPS 40. Question client regarding expectations; explain nature of composites.					
41. Select composite shade, place small amount of material on the tooth near the lesion and cure it; involve client in shade selection.					
42. Place dental dam.					
43. After cavity preparation, apply cavity liner, sealer, and/or base as needed.					
44. Place matrix and wedge to obtain tight seal at gingival margin.					
45. Use forceps to place the bi-tine ring. Ring forceps are designed for and supplied with ring kit. Rubber dam forceps also may be used. The ring can be placed on either side of the wedge, depending on size of the prep. The tines of the ring should be positioned as close as possible to the cavosurface margin to ensure a tight seal.					

Continued

243

Performance Criteria	*	Self	Peer	Instructor	Comments
46. Examine the cavity preparation carefully and develop a mental picture of the outline form of the preparation as well as the anatomy of the adjacent tooth surface. An over-filled restoration can be difficult to finish if you do not remember the location of the cavosurface margins.					
47. Etch, prime, and bond the tooth preparation. Before placement of composite restorative materials, the clinician must etch, prime, and bond the tooth preparation (collectively called *adhesives*). The proper use of adhesives is critical to the success of composite restorations. There are different types, systems, and manufacturers of adhesives (e.g., total etch, prime and bond, all-in-one). Because they are applied in different manners, it is important to follow the directions from the respective manufacturer.					
48. Many clinicians promote the application of a flowable resin to line the floor of the proximal box. There is some evidence that it improves the adaptation of this area and minimizes the potential for voids. The flowable composite is applied by ejecting a small amount across the gingival floor of the preparation. A thickness of only 0.5 mm is needed. After light curing for 20 seconds, the next step is to layer the composite material into the preparation.					
49. Incrementally fill: Composite is added in incremental layers because the light emitted from a curing light can penetrate through only a certain thickness of material. Most curing lights cure to a maximum depth of 2 mm, so small increments are required. Another reason composite is added in thin increments is as composite material sets, it shrinks on a microscopic level. Keeping each layer of composite thin means that the cumulative effects of this distortion will be less problematic than if the composite were placed and cured as a single thick mass. Each layer should be cured for 20 seconds.					
50. Place subsequent layers and shape the anatomy. Depending on the depth of the preparation, a third layer or even a fourth layer may be required. The anatomy is shaped by using appropriate composite instruments. Keeping the tip in the central groove and angling the instrument up to the cavosurface margin, pat/tamp the material in place. Excess material is wiped up and over the cavosurface margin.					
51. Round and contour the height of the marginal ridge. An explorer or paddle-shaped blade can be used to remove excess composite from and around the matrix band. Again, cure the composite for 20 seconds.					
52. Remove the matrix/wedge. After removing the metal matrix band, cure the interproximal area from the buccal and lingual aspects for 20 seconds each. This provides a final cure to ensure that those areas previously shielded by the metal matrix band are cured fully.					

Performance Criteria	*	Self	Peer	Instructor	Comments
53. Finishing and polishing posterior composite resins can be accomplished immediately after polymerization of composite restorations using any of the variety of composite supplies available. Check the proximal area for overhangs, proper contour, and contact. Using light shaving strokes, a gold knife or Bard Parker blade can be used to remove minor overhangs that may remain.					
54. A flame-shaped finishing bur or composite disc can be used to correct overcontoured areas and remove flash in other areas. Polish the entire surface of the restoration with composite polishing points followed by a composite polishing paste in a rubber cup.					
55. Check the proximal contact with floss. If it is too tight, a finishing strip or tapered bur can be used to correct it.					
56. After assessing the restoration, remove the dental dam.					
57. Evaluate the occlusion with articulating paper and adjust as required. If occlusal adjustment is required, re-polish the areas that were adjusted.					
58. Clinician should inform the patient of the following: a. Patient may experience some minor discomfort of the tissues around the restored tooth because of irritation of the gingival wedge and the finishing of the gingival margin area. b. Desiccation of the tooth may make the tooth look lighter, resulting in a temporary mismatch of the composite shade selection. After a few hours the tooth will rehydrate and the composite color will blend with the natural tooth.					
59. Carve away marking spots on the amalgam until centric occlusion is reestablished as it was before the procedure; re-mark the occlusion as necessary, carving away high spots each time with a carver or round bur, if the amalgam has set up.					
60. Prevention of Disease Transmission	*				
ADDITIONAL COMMENTS					

Performance Objective

By following a routine procedure that meets the stated protocols, the student will demonstrate the appropriate technique for **Procedure 39.4 Placing and Finishing a Class III Composite**

Evaluation and Grading Criteria

Instructor will assign grades for each performance criteria.

<u>3</u> Student competently met stated criteria
<u>2</u> Student required minimal assistance to meet criteria
<u>1</u> Student showed uncertainty when attempting criteria
<u>0</u> Student was not prepared and needs to repeat criteria
<u>N/A</u> Student was not evaluated

Performance Standards

Instructor shall identify steps that are critical with an asterisk (*)

Performance Criteria	*	Self	Peer	Instructor	Comments

EQUIPMENT
    Personal protective equipment
    Protective eyewear for patient
    Isolation materials
    Glass ionomer cavity liner or sealer as needed
    Conditioning agent (acid gel)
    Priming agent
    Bonding resin
    Composite
    Resin surface coating
    Matrix system-Sectional matrix system or Tofflemire retainer
      with precontoured band
    Dispensing syringe
    Curing light and protective shields
    Plastic instruments
    Finishing burs and discs
    Articulating paper					

STEPS 61. Question client regarding expectations; explain nature of composites.					
62. Select composite shade, place small amount of material on the tooth near the lesion and cure it; involve client in shade selection.					
63. Place dental dam.					
64. After cavity preparation, apply cavity liner, sealer, and/or base as needed.					
65. Position a clear, plastic matrix strip between the preparation and the adjacent tooth.					

Continued

Performance Criteria	*	Self	Peer	Instructor	Comments
66. Dry tooth and apply etchant to the entire cavity surface according to manufacturer's instructions. Rinse with an air-water spray for at least 15 seconds; dry with forced-air drying. Reposition matrix as necessary; position a wedge interproximally.					
67. Inspect the peripheral etched pattern.					
68. Apply thin coats of primer to etched surfaces according to manufacturer's instructions and lightly dry.					
69. Apply a thin coat of bonding resin to primed surface; spread resin over etched enamel with a small brush or sponge and a gentle stream of air.					
70. Polymerize bonding resin with curing light for 15 to 20 seconds; light wand should be as close as possible without direct contact. Careful inspection of cured bonding resin will reveal a slightly tacky surface. This very thin layer of resin is unable to polymerize completely because of the influence of air. It will polymerize rapidly once covered by composite or a matrix strip and re-exposed to the curing light.					
71. Remove cap from composite dispensing device; express small amount of selected composite onto a small paper pad; replace cap. Many systems are pre-encapsulated.					
72. With a composite placment instrument, or pre-encapsulated mixture placed in dispensing gun, place increment of composite (no more than 2 mm thick) in preparation; adapt to walls and margins; cure this first increment for 20 to 30 seconds.					
73. Continue to add and cure increments, building form to a slight excess in contour. In small cavities final form may be achieved by firmly wrapping clear matrix against tooth and curing through it; remove wedge and matrix.					
74. Contour restoration with finishing burs and discs, exercising care to avoid tooth damage.					
75. Remove the dental dam and check for occlusal prematurities on restoration. Lingual high spots can be reduced carefully with a large, round finishing bur or a football-shaped fine diamond.					
76. Polish accessible parts of restoration with polishing discs; examine gingival sulcus and remove debris.					
77. If desired, apply resin surface coating with a cotton pellet or foam applicator; cure for 10 seconds.					

Performance Criteria	*	Self	Peer	Instructor	Comments
78. Show client finished restoration.					
79. Prevention of Disease Transmission	*				
ADDITIONAL COMMENTS					

Performance Objective

By following a routine procedure that meets the stated protocols, the student will demonstrate the appropriate technique for **Procedure 39.5 Placing a Resin-Modified Glass Ionomer (RMGI) for Class V Restoration**

Evaluation and Grading Criteria

Instructor will assign grades for each performance criteria.

   3 Student competently met stated criteria
   2 Student required minimal assistance to meet criteria
   1 Student showed uncertainty when attempting criteria
   0 Student was not prepared and needs to repeat criteria
N/A Student was not evaluated

Performance Standards

Instructor shall identify steps that are critical with an asterisk (*)

Performance Criteria	*	Self	Peer	Instructor	Comments

EQUIPMENT
    Personal protective equipment
    Protective eyewear for client
    Isolation materials
    RMGI
    Polyacrylic acid/conditioner
    Pumice
    Polishing cup
    Composite placement instruments
    Carving instrument
    Bonding resin
    Special protective varnish
    Curing light and protective shields
    Matrix system					

STEPS 80. Examine lesions; assess need for local anesthetic agent.					
81. Select shade of restorative material to be used.					
82. Place dental dam.					
83. Place gingival retraction cord as needed.					
84. According to manufacturer's instructions, apply conditioner to abrasion lesion (approximately 15 seconds); rinse thoroughly for 15 seconds with a strong air-water spray, and dry lightly, ensuring a moist surface.					
85. Mix glass ionomer according to manufacturer's directions or triturate pre-encapsulated RMGI.					
86. Rapidly fill cavity to slight excess, using a plastic instrument to place material; if desired, position cervical matrix over cavity to hold cement against tooth; light-cure per directions using protective shield.					
87. Remove matrix.					

Continued

251

Performance Criteria	*	Self	Peer	Instructor	Comments
88. Contour restoration with finishing burs and discs take care to avoid damage to tooth root.					
89. Apply thin coat of bonding resin to cement restoration surface and cure resin for 15 to 20 seconds.					
90. Remove dental dam; examine gingival sulcus and remove debris.					
91. Show final result to client.					
92. Prevention of Disease Transmission	*				
ADDITIONAL COMMENTS					

Performance Objective

By following a routine procedure that meets the stated protocols, the student will demonstrate the appropriate technique for **Procedure 39.6 Finishing and Polishing Amalgam Restorations**

Evaluation and Grading Criteria

Instructor will assign grades for each performance criteria.

 3 Student competently met stated criteria
 2 Student required minimal assistance to meet criteria
 1 Student showed uncertainty when attempting criteria
 0 Student was not prepared and needs to repeat criteria
N/A Student was not evaluated

Performance Standards

Instructor shall identify steps that are critical with an asterisk (*)

Performance Criteria	*	Self	Peer	Instructor	Comments
EQUIPMENT 　Personal protective barriers 　Isolation materials 　Finishing burs 　Carving instruments 　Handpiece 　Rubber polishing cups and points (or flour of pumice and polishing powders)					
STEPS 93. Question client regarding occlusion and tooth sensitivity since restoration was placed.					
94. Explain value of polished versus unpolished restoration to the client.					
95. Examine amalgam for burnish marks; adjust occlusion as necessary with a round finishing bur.					
96. Refine occlusal margins with a sharp discoid carver, drawn in shaving strokes parallel to margins.					
97. Using low to moderate speeds and intermittent brief strokes, polish amalgam with abrasive-impregnated rubber cups and points. Begin with most abrasive, end with least abrasive. Maintain wet field during polishing procedures; avoid over polishing established occlusal contacts.					
98. Rinse mouth of debris.					
99. Show client polished restorations.					
ADDITIONAL COMMENTS					

Performance Objective

By following a routine procedure that meets the stated protocols, the student will demonstrate the appropriate technique for **Procedure 39.7 Placing a Stainless Steel Crown**

Evaluation and Grading Criteria

Instructor will assign grades for each performance criteria.

<u>3</u> Student competently met stated criteria
<u>2</u> Student required minimal assistance to meet criteria
<u>1</u> Student showed uncertainty when attempting criteria
<u>0</u> Student was not prepared and needs to repeat criteria
<u>N/A</u> Student was not evaluated

Performance Standards

Instructor shall identify steps that are critical with an asterisk (*)

Performance Criteria	*	Self	Peer	Instructor	Comments

EQUIPMENT
   Personal protective equipment
   Protective eyewear for client
   Isolation materials
   Stainless steel preformed crowns
   Crown trimming scissors
   Crimping pliers
   Resin-modified glass ionomer cement
   Floss
   Articulating paper					

STEPS 1. Evaluate prepared tooth for size.					
2. Correct size is selected by measuring the mesiodistal width between contact points of a matching tooth in mouth.					
3. Choose smallest crown that will fit.					
4. To seat, place crown lingually and adapt it over the occlusal and buccal aspects of prepared tooth.					
5. Use firm pressure to seat crown. May hear an audible click as it springs over gingival undercut area of preparation.					
6. To evaluate fit, observe marginal gingiva. It will blanch somewhat with a well-fitting crown. If excess blanching is observed, crown will have to be trimmed.					
7. In a properly seated crown, margin should extend approximately 1 mm subgingivally. To trim crown, scribe a line where marginal gingival hits crown with an explorer.					
8. Trim crown 1 mm below scribed line. Use crown scissors or an abrasive wheel to trim crown.					

Continued

Performance Criteria	*	Self	Peer	Instructor	Comments
9. Use crimping pliers to adapt edge of crown for a tighter fit.					
10. Seat crown once more to evaluate fit.					
11. Crown is now ready to be cemented.					
12. Use resin-modified glass ionomer cement. Fill entire crown with cement.					
13. Excess cement will flow out from margins as crown is seated.					
14. Use an explorer, a scaler, and knotted floss to remove excess cement.					
15. Check occlusion using articulating paper.					
16. Infection control	*				
ADDITIONAL COMMENTS					

Performance Objective

By following a routine procedure that meets the stated protocols, the student will demonstrate the appropriate technique for **Procedure 39.9 Placing Gingival Retraction Cord**

Evaluation and Grading Criteria

Instructor will assign grades for each performance criteria.

3 Student competently met stated criteria
2 Student required minimal assistance to meet criteria
1 Student showed uncertainty when attempting criteria
0 Student was not prepared and needs to repeat criteria
N/A Student was not evaluated

Performance Standards

Instructor shall identify steps that are critical with an asterisk (*)

Performance Criteria	*	Self	Peer	Instructor	Comments
EQUIPMENT Personal protective equipment Protective eyewear for client Examination kit (mouth mirror, explorer, periodontal probe, cotton pliers) Dappen dish Scissors 2 × 2 gauze Cotton rolls or dry angles Retraction cord hemostatic agent Retraction cord of various sizes Astringent and coagulation liquid					
STEPS 1. Estimate circumference of preparation; cut a piece of bottom cord to encompass preparation margins.					
2. Cut a piece of top cord that is approximately ½ inch longer than bottom cord and thicker in diameter. The top cord is longer and thicker than the bottom cord because it provides primary lateral tissue displacement necessary for satisfactorily allowing injection of impression material.					
3. Soak bottom and top cords in hemostatic agent; place cord on a dry 2 × 2 gauze to remove excess solution.					
4. Isolate site with cotton rolls and/or dry angles.					
5. Using bottom cord, lasso tooth with loop around lingual aspect of the tooth.					
6. Start placement of bottom cord in one of the interproximal areas using a periodontal probe; while periodontal probe holds packed cord in place, side of the explorer rotates the cord into sulcus. Cord placement is achieved by gently rolling cord down tooth into the gingival sulcus and below gingival margin of the preparation. Avoid forceful apical pressure on cord.					

Continued

Performance Criteria	*	Self	Peer	Instructor	Comments
7. Proceed in a methodic manner around the tooth, ending on the facial surface. Work from one end of cord to other; avoid skipping around. Excess cord should be cut at this point to avoid overlapping.					
8. With bottom cord in place, take top cord and lasso tooth, with loop around the lingual aspect of tooth.					
9. Start placement of top cord in one of the interproximal areas; proceed with placement technique described in steps 6 and 7. Depending on the gingival status, the top cord placement may not be below the gingival margin of the preparation. A small end of the top cord will extend out of the sulcus after it has been placed around circumference of tooth.					
10. Infection control	*				
ADDITIONAL COMMENTS					

Performance Objective

By following a routine procedure that meets the stated protocols, the student will demonstrate the appropriate technique for **Procedure 39.9 Preparing Reinforced Zinc Oxide and Eugenol Temporary Restoration**

Evaluation and Grading Criteria

Instructor will assign grades for each performance criteria.

    <u>3</u> Student competently met stated criteria
    <u>2</u> Student required minimal assistance to meet criteria
    <u>1</u> Student showed uncertainty when attempting criteria
    <u>0</u> Student was not prepared and needs to repeat criteria
<u>N/A</u> Student was not evaluated

Performance Standards

Instructor shall identify steps that are critical with an asterisk (*)

Performance Criteria	*	Self	Peer	Instructor	Comments

EQUIPMENT
    Personal protective equipment
    Protective eyewear for client
    Isolation materials
    Tofflemire matrix system
    Petrolatum
    Reinforced zinc oxide and eugenol
    Nonabsorbent mixing pad
    Plastic instruments
    Cotton pellets and rolls, dry aids
    Finishing burs
    Carving instruments
    Articulating paper					

STEPS 11. Isolate operating site as appropriate.					
12. Prepare Tofflemire matrix system. Apply thin coat of petrolatum on the inside of the matrix band; position matrix, secure it, and place interproximal wedges as needed.					
13. Use manufacturer's instructions for measuring and mixing. Premeasured capsules are available and are mixed with a triturator.					
14. Prepare mix; when material reaches consistency of firm clay, carry an ample amount to cavity with a plastic instrument. Firmly adapt rubbery material to all walls of cavity with a placement instrument.					
15. Fill cavity to slight excess; shape occlusal anatomy by using a moist cotton pellet in cotton forceps to create a general anatomic form.					
16. When material has hardened, remove wedge(s), retainer, and matrix band; apply pressure apically on the temporary restoration to counteract removal of band.					

Continued

Performance Criteria	*	Self	Peer	Instructor	Comments
17. Check proximal and gingival margins for excess material and remove with sharp, narrow-bladed carving instrument.					
18. Remove isolation materials; evaluate premature occlusion on temporary restoration with articulating paper and adjust as necessary with large, round bur and carving instruments.					
19. Examine gingival sulcus for debris and remove as necessary; excess material at gingival margin can be removed using a bladed instrument such as the ½ Hollenbeck or IPC carver.					
20. Infection control	*				
ADDITIONAL COMMENTS					

40 Orthodontic Care

COMPETENCIES

1. Discuss malocclusion, including the effects of malocclusion.
2. Assess and evaluate the need for a referral for orthodontic care.
3. Educate patients and guardians to understand normal developmental changes versus orthodontic needs, and describe various orthodontic considerations that affect dental care.
4. Describe the biomechanics of tooth movement.
5. List and describe the three types of orthodontic treatment.
6. Detail the uses of a variety of orthodontic appliances.
7. Identify risks associated with orthodontic treatment and communicate how to mitigate or manage the risks.
8. Discuss the need for dental collaboration when dealing with alternative orthodontic treatment to address restorative, periodontal, and implant needs.
9. Instruct patients on effective self-care regimens to address hard and soft tissue concerns during treatment.

SHORT ANSWER QUESTIONS

1. What is held in place by brackets that are bonded to the teeth and held in place by a ligature?

   _____

   _____

   _____

2. What are bonded to teeth to hold archwires?

   _____

   _____

   _____

3. What are small ties or rings that can be made of elastic or wire?

   _____

   _____

   _____

4. What type of appliance holds maxillary molars in place to hold their position?

   _____

   _____

   _____

5. What is a permanent stainless steel wire bonded to lingual surfaces of teeth to aid in holding tooth position?

   _____

   _____

   _____

6. List additional assessment data the dental hygienist may collect on patients with orthodontics.

_____

_____

_____

_____

7. List oral hygiene interventions the dental hygienist may utilizefor patients with orthodontics.

_____

_____

_____

_____

_____

_____

_____

FILL IN THE BLANK STATEMENTS

Select the best term from the chapter and complete the following statements.

1. Phase I orthodontics is also known as _____.

2. Phase 2 orthodontics is also known as _____.

3. _____ may occur under or adjacent to orthodontic bands and brackets.

4. _____ examine peri-oral structures for pathology, supernumerary teeth, congenitally missing teeth, and impacted teeth.

5. _____ are a sequence of trays that apply pressure similar to the action of, and may be used in lieu of, the archwire and brackets.

MULTIPLE CHOICE QUESTIONS

Complete each question by circling the best answer.

1. An orthodontic examination is recommended for children by the age of 7 due to all of the following reasons EXCEPT:
   a. Basic occlusal relationship with first permanent molars can be established
   b. Jaw discrepancies can be evaluated
   c. Beginning long-term orthodontic is recommended to prevent future malocclusion
   d. Early interceptive therapy demonstrates effective outcomes

2. Malocclusion can occur in all of the following planes EXCEPT:
   a. Lateral
   b. Sagittal
   c. Transverse
   d. Occlusal

3. All of the following conditions are reasons for an orthodontic consult EXCEPT:
   a. Early loss of primary teeth
   b. Retention of primary teeth
   c. Crowding
   d. High caries rate

4. All of the following extra-oral photos are standard for orthodontic evaluation EXCEPT:
   a. Full-face smiling
   b. Full-face frowning
   c. Profile smiling
   d. Profile not smiling

5. Most orthodontists prefer to start orthodontic treatment during teen years. Teens have rapid bone growth rates.
   a. Both statements are true.
   b. Both statements are false.
   c. The first statement is true, the second statement is false.
   d. The first statement is false, the second statement is true.

6. The goal of orthopedic expansion is to:
   a. Reduce the need for extracting permanent teeth
   b. Increase arch length by tipping teeth facially
   c. Decrease arch length by tipping teeth lingually
   d. Retain primate spaces through age 7

7. Midline diastemas of 2-3 mm or more may be caused by all of the following EXCEPT:
   a. Missing lateral incisors
   b. High frenal attachment
   c. Supernumerary tooth at the midline
   d. Tooth size discrepancy

8. Dental age is the maturation of teeth and clinical eruption pattern. Skeletal stage is the patients' age in years and months.
   a. Both statements are true.
   b. Both statements are false.
   c. The first statement is true, the second statement is false.
   d. The first statement is false, the second statement is true.

9. Cone beam computed tomography produces 3D images of teeth, soft tissue, nerve, and bone. Lateral cephalometric image assesses facial and jaw proportions.
   a. Both statements are true.
   b. Both statements are false.
   c. The first statement is true, the second statement is false.
   d. The first statement is false, the second statement is true.

10. A thin plastic retainer that fully covers all maxillary teeth that retains movement and prevents relapse is:
    a. Plastic tray aligner
    b. Essix retainer
    c. Hawley appliance
    d. Head gear

11. All of the following are reasons for referral for orthodontic treatment EXCEPT:
    a. Improve facial esthetics
    b. Evaluate patterns of growth and development
    c. Evaluate malocclusion
    d. Decrease caries risk

12. All of the following are possible negative outcomes of rapid orthodontic movement EXCEPT:
    a. Apical root resorption
    b. Gingival overgrowth
    c. Recession
    d. Bone loss

CASE STUDY

Your 15-year-old male patient reports to your office for routine dental hygiene care. He is full orthodontic therapy with bands on molars and brackets on all other teeth. His last dental hygiene appointment was 6 months ago.

Extra and intraoral findings include:

- Generalized severe marginal gingival inflammation with some areas of hyperplasia
- Moderate to heavy biofilm generalized
- Signs of demineralization around buccal surfaces of all teeth
- Probe readings are >3 mm generalized

Patient reports brushing 4-5 times a week, not flossing, diet high in sugar.

1. What education plan do you present to your patient?
2. What interventions do you recommend?
3. When should this patient return for further dental hygiene services?
4. What dietary counseling do you recommend?
5. What Human Needs Model deficits does this patient present with?

_____

_____

_____

_____

_____

_____

_____

_____

_____

_____

_____

_____

41 Fixed and Removable Dental Prostheses

SHORT ANSWER QUESTIONS

1. List the risk factors for tooth loss.

_____

_____

_____

_____

2. Name eight factors that contribute to xerostomia.

_____

_____

_____

_____

_____

_____

_____

3. Describe the treatment for chronic candidiasis.

_____

_____

_____

_____

_____

4. Why are regular maintenance appointments still advised for the fully edentulous patient?

_____

_____

_____

_____

5. What are the causes of denture stomatitis?

_____

_____

_____

_____

_____

_____

_____

FILL IN THE BLANK STATEMENTS

Select the best term from the chapter and complete the following statements.

1. _____ reduces stability on retention prostheses.

2. The artificial tooth that occupies edentulous space is a _____.

3. An _____ is a tooth or implant used to connect the
_____.

4. _____ is inflammation of oral mucosa underneath a denture that includes erythema, pain, and swelling.

5. _____ is abnormal gingival tissue growth due to irritation from a denture.

MULTIPLE CHOICE QUESTIONS

Complete each question by circling the best answer.

1. All of the following conditions contribute to mandibular atrophy EXCEPT:
   a. Diabetes
   b. Metabolic bone disease
   c. Diet low in calcium
   d. Post-menopausal osteoporosis

2. Bony changes in maxillary and mandibular arches differ significantly. Mandibular bone resorbs four times greater than maxillary bone.
   a. Both statements are true.
   b. Both statements are false.
   c. The first statement is true, the second statement is false.
   d. The first statement is false, the second statement is true.

3. Patients with removable partial dentures have 20% chewing efficiency as compared to those with natural teeth. Decreased chewing efficiency is due to loss of gingival support.
   a. Both statements are true.
   b. Both statements are false.
   c. The first statement is true, the second statement is false.
   d. The first statement is false, the second statement is true.

4. Which drug prescription category may increase salivary flow?
   a. Calcium channel blocker
   b. Beta blocker
   c. Diuretics
   d. Cholinergics

5. All of the following are characteristics of angular cheilitis EXCEPT:
   a. Pain
   b. Vitamin B deficiency
   c. Caused by *Streptococcus sanguini*
   d. Loss of vertical dimension

6. Characteristics of chronic candidiasis include all of the following EXCEPT:
   a. Poor denture occlusion
   b. Affects mandibular mucosal tissues more than maxillary
   c. Poor biofilm removal
   d. Diabetes

7. Tooth loss can impact all of the following oral changes EXCEPT:
   a. Fear of aging
   b. Residual ridge resorption
   c. Loss of orofacial muscle tone
   d. Mucous membrane remodeling

8. A hard acrylic appliance that fits over natural teeth to create a functional occlusion is:
   a. Obturator
   b. Athletic mouth guard
   c. Bruxism guard
   d. Partial denture

9. An appliance designed to cover an opening in the oral cavity to prevent food or fluids from entering the nasal passages is:
   a. Obturator
   b. Athletic mouth guard
   c. Bruxism guard
   d. Partial denture

10. Which of the following is not a cause of xerostomia?
    a. Multiple medications
    b. Diabetes
    c. Candidiasis
    d. Age

11. A bridge is also known as:
    a. Crown
    b. Restoration
    c. Fixed partial denture
    d. Acrylic flipper

12. All of the following are symptoms of xerostomia EXCEPT:
    a. Candidiasis
    b. Burning mouth syndrome
    c. Speech difficulties
    d. Altered taste

CASE STUDY

Your 70-year-old male patient reports for routine dental hygiene therapy. He has a full maxillary acrylic denture and a removable mandibular partial denture that has metal clasps.

Extra- and intraoral clinical exam findings:

- Angular cheilitis and ulcerations of the lips
- Heavy biofilm on both dentures and around remaining teeth
- Shiny erythematous tissue on palate
- Generalized pocket depths 1-2 mm with 1-mm recession facial and lingual with moderate BOP
- Slight supragingival calculus lingually
- Mandibular denture has one broken clasp
- Patient reports pain when chewing

1. What Human Needs Conceptual model deficits does this patient present with?
2. What education topics would you cover?
3. What will you recommend for the patient's broken clasp?
4. How would you further investigate his pain?
5. What dental prostheses cleansing products would you recommend?
6. What nutritional recommendations would you make for your patient?
7. What interval of dental hygiene services would you recommend to this patient?

_____

_____

_____

_____

_____

_____

_____

_____

_____

_____

_____

_____

_____

_____

Performance Objective

By following a routine procedure that meets the stated protocols, the student will demonstrate the appropriate technique for **41-1 Professional Care for Patients With Removable Dental Prostheses**

Evaluation and Grading Criteria

Instructor will assign grades for each performance criteria.

<u>3</u> Student competently met stated criteria
<u>2</u> Student required minimal assistance to meet criteria
<u>1</u> Student showed uncertainty when attempting criteria
<u>0</u> Student was not prepared and needs to repeat criteria
<u>N/A</u> Student was not evaluated

Performance Standards

Instructor shall identify steps that are critical with an asterisk (*)

Performance Criteria	*	Self	Peer	Instructor	Comments

EQUIPMENT
  Protective barriers
  Prophy cup and bristled brush
  Low-speed hand piece
  Antimicrobial mouth rinse
  Tin oxide
  Mouth mirror
  Hand mirror
  Gauze
  Tongue blades
  Small plastic bag
  Stain and calculus remover solution
  Ultrasonic cleaning unit					

STEPS					
1. Update patient's health history to identify systemic disorders, current medications, and conditions that may affect care and ability to wear the prostheses.					
2. Review patient's personal history records; note details such as age, occupation, and culture.					
3. Review patient's dental history.					
4. Ask patient to explain prostheses problems experienced; listen attentively to complaints.					
5. Perform comprehensive assessment of head and neck.					
6. Assess the temporomandibular joint (TMJ) and associated musculature as patient opens and closes mouth and slides jaw from side to side.					
7. Assess extra-oral soft tissues.					
8. Assess intraoral soft tissues for evidence of local denture trauma or systemic diseases, and record lesion color, texture, size, contour, and presence of pain.					

Continued

269

Performance Criteria	*	Self	Peer	Instructor	Comments
9. Visually inspect the prosthesis for cleanliness and palpate prosthesis-bearing mucosa with prosthesis out of the mouth.					
10. Assess the structure and form of the alveolar ridges.					
11. Document changes in associated structures, including the tongue, floor of the mouth, and oropharynx.					
12. Assess oral hygiene status.					
13. Ask patient to displace the prosthesis away from supporting tissues. The posterior border seal of the maxillary denture is checked by attempting to pull the anterior teeth forward.					
14. Assess stability of the prosthesis with respect to its position during normal oral functions.					
15. Indicate changes in occlusion and articulation.					
16. Analyze objective and subjective assessment data.					
17. Present significant findings to patient and dentist.					
18. Determine a dental-hygiene care plan and goals to be achieved in consultation with patient and dentist.					
19. Review self-care and dental care; suggest methods for improvement.					
20. Counsel patient on adequate nutrition.					
21. Fill a small plastic bag with cleaning solution, label with patient's name, submerge the prosthesis in it, and place the bag in an ultrasonic cleaning unit.					
22. Lightly polish the prosthesis with an extremely fine polishing agent (tin oxide) *on external surfaces only,* and thoroughly rinse under warm water (when appropriate).					
23. Discuss continued-care interval. Emphasize the importance of regular professional care.					
24. Measure the achievement of goals established at the previous dental hygiene care appointment.					
25. Formulate an evaluative statement regarding the level of goal attainment.					

Performance Criteria	*	Self	Peer	Instructor	Comments
26. Document service in patient's record under "Services Rendered" and date entry.					
27. Prevention of Disease Transmission	*				
ADDITIONAL COMMENTS					

Performance Objective

By following a routine procedure that meets the stated protocols, the student will demonstrate the appropriate technique for **41-2 Daily Oral and Denture Hygiene Care for Individuals With Removable Prostheses**

Evaluation and Grading Criteria

Instructor will assign grades for each performance criteria.

3 Student competently met stated criteria
2 Student required minimal assistance to meet criteria
1 Student showed uncertainty when attempting criteria
0 Student was not prepared and needs to repeat criteria
N/A Student was not evaluated

Performance Standards

Instructor shall identify steps that are critical with an asterisk (*)

Performance Criteria	*	Self	Peer	Instructor	Comments

EQUIPMENT
   Soft denture brush, soft intraoral toothbrush, antimicrobial mouth rinse
   Basin
   Denture cup
   Towel
   Dilute sodium hypochlorite solution (removable complete dentures) or commercial denture cleanser (removable partial dentures and implant supported dentures)
   Warm water
   Wall-mounted mirror
   Soft nylon toothbrush					

STEPS 28. Explain the importance of daily care for both dentures and soft tissues.					
29. Describe the consequences of oral and denture hygiene neglect.					
30. Summarize the patient's responsibilities in monitoring oral function and health status.					
31. Advise against the use of denture home repair kits and encourage the patient to return to the dentist for proper care.					
32. Discourage use of denture adhesives with a stable and retentive prosthesis. Under dentist supervision, a small amount of adhesive (3-4 pea-sized drops) may be applied to the inner surface that directly contacts the oral mucosa. Denture adhesives are not normally used with partial removable dentures.					
33. Remind the patient to brush dentures after each meal and before going to bed or, at the very least, to rinse it under running water.					

Continued

273

Performance Criteria	*	Self	Peer	Instructor	Comments
34. Teach self-examination of denture for proper fit, denture deposits, and abraded inner and outer surfaces.					
35. Teach patient that some commercially available denture powders and pastes are too abrasive for dentures and are not recommended for use.					
36. Suggest daily use of fresh denture immersion cleansers. Recommend a diluted sodium hypochlorite solution as a cleanser for complete dentures. Soak complete dentures for 5 to 10 minutes, and rinse thoroughly. Partial dentures benefit from alkaline peroxide solutions found in many denture-cleansing products, usually in the form of a tablet. Soak partial denture for 15 minutes or overnight, and rinse thoroughly. Change solutions daily.					
37. Teach the patient to remove denture when possible and at night while at rest.					
38. Assemble supplies.					
39. Fill basin with water and line with a small towel.					
40. Gently remove denture and rinse away saliva and loose debris. In the case of complete dentures, remove any denture adhesive material.					
41. Firmly grasp denture in palm of one hand and hold over water-filled basin.					
42. Demonstrate use of a denture brush with a mild soap solution or nonabrasive denture paste to remove accumulations on the inner impression and outer polished surfaces, and adapt brush as necessary.					
43. Rinse denture and brush under running water to completely remove all denture cleanser.					
44. Inspect denture for any remaining biofilm, food debris, or cleanser by visual and tactile examination.					
45. Place prosthesis in a denture cup.					
46. On removal of denture, rinse mouth with warm water, antimicrobial mouth rinse, or saline solution.					
47. Teach patient to use a soft toothbrush or soft cloth daily to clean edentulous mucosa and tongue by employing long strokes in a posterior-to-anterior direction.					

Performance Criteria	*	Self	Peer	Instructor	Comments
48. Teach patient to use thumb and index finger to massage edentulous tissues daily by applying pressure and then releasing it continually along the ridge. Mechanical, vibratory stimulation with the sides of multi-tufted soft toothbrush filaments can provide similar results.					
49. Prevention of Disease Transmission	*				
ADDITIONAL COMMENTS					

42 Dentinal Hypersensitivity

COMPETENCIES

1. Distinguish between dentinal hypersensitivity and other sources of tooth pain.
2. Discuss oral conditions associated with dentinal hypersensitivity, elucidate the teeth and risk factors most likely contributing to dentinal hypersensitivity, and describe the prevalence and distribution of dentinal hypersensitivity.
3. Explain the specific clinical and radiographic criteria that must be present to arrive at a diagnosis of dentinal hypersensitivity.
4. Describe the management of dentinal hypersensitivity, including the indications and effectiveness of various treatment options.

SHORT ANSWER QUESTIONS

1. List characteristic of dentinal hypersensitivity.

_____

_____

_____

_____

_____

_____

_____

_____

2. List causes of gingival recession that may contribute to dentinal hypersensitivity.

_____

_____

_____

_____

_____

_____

_____

_____

_____

_____

_____

3. List toothbrush conditions that contribute to abrasion.

_____

_____

_____

_____

_____

_____

_____

_____

_____

_____

_____

4. List recommendations for managing hypersensitivity.

_____

_____

_____

_____

_____

_____

5. List treatment options for dentinal hypersensitivity.

_____

_____

_____

_____

6. Give examples of chemicals available that seal dentinal tubules.

7. List factors that contribute to dentinal hypersensitivity.

FILL IN THE BLANK STATEMENTS

Select the best term from the chapter and complete the following statements.

1. _____ is an exaggerated sharp pain response to application of stimuli to exposed dentin that cannot be attributed to any other form of dental defect or pathology.

2. _____ are composed of small myelinated fibers that induce a sensation of localized sharp pain and are thought to be responsible for dentinal hypersensitivity.

3. _____ respond sensitively to electrical stimulation.

4. _____ cause a dull, poorly localized, aching type of pain usually associated with pulpal pain.

5. _____ covers and protects the opening of the dentinal tubules or mineral compounds obstruct the tubules from stimulating nerve conduction to the pulp.

6. _____ suggests that painful stimuli are transmitted to the pulp surface via movement of fluid found within the dentinal tubules.

7. _____ uses low-amperage direct electrical current to introduce ionized substances into dentinal tissues.

MULTIPLE CHOICE QUESTIONS

Complete each question by circling the best answer.

1. All the following products have weak or limited research supporting desensitizing effectiveness EXCEPT:
   a. Stannous fluoride 0.4%
   b. Potassium nitrate 5%
   c. Oxalates
   d. Casein

2. Bulimia may cause what type of erosion?
   a. Intrinsic
   b. Primary
   c. Extrinsic
   d. Secondary

3. All of the following are true concerning 38% silver diamide fluoride EXCEPT:
   a. FDA approved for caries prevention
   b. Stains active carious lesions black
   c. Uses iontophoresis as method of action
   d. Effective desensitizing agent

4. All of the following clinical criteria must be met to reach a diagnosis of dental hypersensitivity EXCEPT:
   a. No caries
   b. No fractures
   c. Sensitivity to stimuli
   d. Exposed cementum at the site of sensitivity

5. Strontium acetate is a bonding resin to seal and desensitize nerves within dentinal tubules. Glutaraldehyde chemically blocks open dentinal tubules.
   a. Both statements are true.
   b. Both statements are false.
   c. The first statement is true and the second statement is false.
   d. The first statement is false and the second statement is true.

6. The most common cementum-to-enamel relationship is:
   a. Enamel overlaps cementum
   b. Cementum and enamel do not meet
   c. Cementum and enamel meet without overlap
   d. Cementum overlaps enamel

7. The physiologically progressive loss of hard tooth structure caused by mastication or grinding between opposing teeth is:
   a. Abrasion
   b. Abfraction
   c. Attrition
   d. Primary erosion

8. Your patient presents with multiple facial areas of severe recession and complains of dentinal sensitivity. She also has several areas of active caries and moderate biofilm generalized. Her last dental appointment was 3 years ago. What is the first Human Needs Conceptual model deficit to address?
   a. Freedom from Pain
   b. Skin and Mucous Membrane Integrity of the Head and Neck
   c. Biologically Sound and Functional Dentition
   d. Responsibility for Oral Health

9. Excessive consumption of carbonated sugar drinks may cause what type of erosion?
   a. Intrinsic
   b. Primary
   c. Extrinsic
   d. Secondary

10. Non-carious lesions caused by occlusal forces are called:
    a. Erosion
    b. Abfraction
    c. Attrition
    d. Abrasion

11. Vital teeth bleaching using peroxides is a common side effect of dentinal hypersensitivity. Gingival recession following surgical periodontal therapy always causes dentinal hypersensitivity.
    a. Both statements are true.
    b. Both statements are false.
    c. The first statement is true and the second statement is false.
    d. The first statement is false and the second statement is true.

12. All of the following radiographic findings must be confirmed to clinically exclude caries EXCEPT:
    a. No fracture lines
    b. No radiolucency at cervical third of tooth
    c. No radiolucent areas under restorations
    d. No apical pathology

13. Which sensory fibers are most likely responsible for dentinal hypersensitivity?
    a. Sharpey's fibers
    b. A-delta fibers
    c. A-beta fibers
    d. C-fibers

14. The most common teeth that experience gingival recession area:
    a. Maxillary anterior
    b. Maxillary posterior
    c. Mandibular anterior
    d. Mandibular posterior

15. The most common teeth surfaces that experience dentinal hypersensitivity are:
    a. Facial
    b. Incisal
    c. Lingual
    d. Occlusal

CASE STUDY MR. EXMORE

Mr. Exmore is a married father of three girls (ages 4, 7, and 10). He has a very stressful job as an air traffic controller. He has been a patient of yours for 3 years and sees you every 6 months for routine dental hygiene care. He uses a hard toothbrush and reports brushing 5-6 times a day with whitening toothpaste. He flosses twice a day and states that he does not like anything stuck in his teeth.

1. Would you and the dentist diagnose Mr. Exmore with dentinal hypersensitivity? Why?
2. What specific home care direction would you give?
3. What are your treatment options?
4. Speculate as to why he has gingival recession.
5. Create a Human Needs Conceptual Model for Mr. Exmore.

_____

_____

_____

_____

_____

_____

_____

_____

Age	38	SCENARIO
Gender	M	**EOE/IOE:**
Height	6'1"	Within normal limits
Weight	220 lb	Slight calculus supragingival on mandibular anterior teeth
B/P	160/100 mm Hg	Localized attrition on all anterior teeth
Chief Complaint	My teeth are very sensitive to cold drinks and certain foods.	**Periodontal Findings:** Probing depths of 1-2 mm generalized
Medical History	Anxiety, OCD	Minimal BOP Generalized recession 2-3 mm on labial surfaces of all anterior teeth, 3-4 mm all posterior teeth on the facial surfaces
Current Medications	Paxil	Abfraction on all maxillary premolars and molars
Social History		**Radiographic Findings:** Incipient carious lesion #12 distal and #13 mesial
		Dental Findings: No caries clinically visible

Using the data from this patient, develop a Human Needs Conceptual model for treatment.

Dental Hygiene Diagnosis (unmet human need)	Etiology (due to…)	Signs and Symptoms (evidenced by…)	Patient Goals (expected outcomes)
Protection from Health Risks			
Freedom from Fear and Stress			
Freedom from Pain			
Wholesome Facial Image			
Skin and Mucous Membrane Integrity of the Head and Neck			
Biologically Sound and Functional Dentition			
Conceptualization and Problem Solving			
Responsibility for Oral Health			

Performance Objective

By following a routine procedure that meets the stated protocols, the student will demonstrate the appropriate technique for **Procedure 42-1 Administration of Desensitizing Agents**

Evaluation and Grading Criteria

Instructor will assign grades for each performance criteria.

    3 Student competently met stated criteria
    2 Student required minimal assistance to meet criteria
    1 Student showed uncertainty when attempting criteria
    0 Student was not prepared and needs to repeat criteria
N/A Student was not evaluated

Performance Standards

Instructor shall identify steps that are critical with an asterisk (*)

Performance Criteria	*	Self	Peer	Instructor	Comments
EQUIPMENT ■ Isolating materials (cotton rolls, gauze, or dry angles) ■ Cotton applicators ■ Dappen dish ■ Personal protective equipment ■ Desensitizing agent					
STEPS 1. Assemble armamentarium for desensitization.					
2. Explain rationale, procedure, and limitations of desensitizing agent to client.					
3. Identify sensitive sites requiring desensitization treatment.					
4. Remove oral biofilm and debris from tooth surfaces before desensitizing agent is applied.					
5. Isolate area with cotton rolls, and dry dentin surface by blotting with gauze.					
6. Dispense desensitizing agent and apply according to manufacturer's instructions.					
7. Evaluate treated areas for success; reapply if necessary.					
8. Discard materials according to infection control procedures.					
9. Record treatment in services-rendered section of dental record, including tooth number, region of treatment, agent used, and patient response.					
10. Educate patient about supplementary procedures for controlling sensitivity.					

Continued

Performance Criteria	*	Self	Peer	Instructor	Comments
11. Prevention of Disease Transmission	*				
ADDITIONAL COMMENTS					

43 Local Anesthesia

COMPETENCIES

1. Discuss the physiologic mechanism of nerve conduction and the primary action of local anesthetics as it relates to pain management and patient comfort.
2. Evaluate various topical and local anesthetic agents and their indications/contraindications for safe and effective use.
3. Describe the local anesthetic armamentarium components, including the procedures for appropriate setup and breakdown.
4. Determine anatomical landmarks, nerves, and areas anesthetized after applying safe and effective procedural techniques for each injection.
5. Describe various local and systemic complications that may develop despite pre-anesthetic patient assessment and adherence to recommended procedures for local anesthesia administration.

SHORT ANSWER QUESTIONS

1. List ideal properties of a local anesthetic.

_____

_____

_____

_____

_____

_____

_____

_____

_____

_____

_____

_____

_____

_____

_____

_____

_____

_____

_____

2. What are the four ways a local anesthetic interferes with pain.

_____

_____

_____

_____

_____

_____

3. What are the advantages of the computer-controlled LA delivery system?

_____

_____

_____

_____

_____

_____

_____

_____

_____

_____

4. List the various stimuli that that change the ion balance if a nerve fiber.

_____

_____

_____

_____

_____

_____

_____

_____

5. How does vasoconstriction impact local anesthesia?

_____

_____

_____

_____

_____

_____

_____

_____

_____

_____

_____

6. What are the generic names/proprietary names of the amides?

_____

_____

_____

_____

_____

_____

_____

7. List health conditions that require special consideration prior to administering local anesthesia.

_____

_____

_____

_____

_____

_____

_____

_____

8. List how vasoconstrictors affect local anesthesia?

_____

_____

_____

_____

_____

9. What phase of conduction do local anesthetics have their primary effect?

_____

_____

_____

10. What causes paresthesia?

_____

_____

_____

_____

_____

_____

_____

_____

FILL IN THE BLANK STATEMENTS

Select the best term from the chapter and complete the following statements.

1. _____ is the most common injectable local anesthetic used in dentistry.

2. _____ is the angled point of the needle that is directed into the tissues.

3. _____ is when the ion balance of the nerve cells reverses, allowing interior nerve to be positively charged.

4. _____ is the most common vasoconstrictor added to local anesthesia.

5. _____ is the most common topical anesthetic agent and is rarely used as an injectable agent.

6. _____ deposits the solution near large terminal nerve branches, and a nerve block involves the deposition of solution close to a main nerve trunk, often at some distance from the treatment area.

7. _____ is part of an aspirating syringe used to imbed into the rubber stopper of the liquid anesthetic cartridge for aspiration.

8. _____ is when blood has escaped from ruptured capillaries and is interspersed into surrounding tissue, usually due to trauma.

9. _____ is the temporary loss of sensation in a specific part of the body by injecting an agent without inducing loss of consciousness.

10. _____ is an amide topical anesthetic 2.5% lidocaine and 2.5% prilocaine used for local anesthesia.

11. _____ is when the nerve is polarized.

12. _____ agents are drugs that constrict the blood vessels and thus control blood flow in the area of the injection.

13. _____ is relaxation of the blood vessel wall resulting in increased blood flow to the injection site.

Complete each question by circling the best answer.

1. All of the following are appropriate injections for maxillary anesthesia EXCEPT:
   a. ASA
   b. Greater palatine
   c. MSA
   d. Gow Gates

2. All of the following are components of nerve conduction EXCEPT:
   a. Membrane is potential
   b. Resting potential is a negative potential
   c. Interior of the nerve is positive in relation to exterior
   d. An electrical charge exists across the membrane

3. Local anesthetic agents interfere with excitation process in the nerve membrane via any of the following EXCEPT:
   a. Altering the threshold potential
   b. Prolonging the rate of depolarization
   c. Increasing the rate of depolarization
   d. Altering the basic resting potential of the nerve membrane

4. Local anesthetic agents cross the blood-brain barrier. Local anesthetics do not cross the placenta.
   a. Both statements are true.
   b. Both statements are false.
   c. The first statement is true and the second statement is false.
   d. The first statement is false and the second statement is true.

5. The best injection type that will provide profound anesthesia to #22-24 is:
   a. IA
   b. Gow Gates
   c. Incisive nerve block
   d. Long buccal nerve block

6. Sensory neurons transmit sensation (pain) toward the brain with the cell body on the end. Motor neurons carry impulses away from the brain (CNS) to the periphery with their cell body between the axon and dendrites.
   a. Both statements are true.
   b. Both statements are false.
   c. The first statement is true and the second statement is false.
   d. The first statement is false and the second statement is true.

7. A relative contraindication to local anesthesia means that the drug in question may be administered to the patient after careful weighing of the risk of using the drug against its potential benefit, and if an acceptable alternative drug is not available. An absolute contraindication does not allow the administration of the drug under any circumstances.
   a. Both statements are true.
   b. Both statements are false.
   c. The first statement is true and the second statement is false.
   d. The first statement is false and the second statement is true.

8. Local anesthesia agents block or inhibit sodium channels and prevent sodium ions from passing through the membrane. This inhibits the depolarization effect and does not conduct the stimulus.
   a. Both statements are true.
   b. Both statements are false.
   c. The first statement is true and the second statement is false.
   d. The first statement is false and the second statement is true.

9. The primary excretory organs for amides local anesthetics are the kidneys. Amides are contraindicated for patients with renal disease.
   a. Both statements are true.
   b. Both statements are false.
   c. The first statement is true and the second statement is false.
   d. The first statement is false and the second statement is true.

10. A hematoma is more likely to develop after a palatal injection. Trismus and pain are common with a hematoma.
    a. Both statements are true.
    b. Both statements are false.
    c. The first statement is true and the second statement is false.
    d. The first statement is false and the second statement is true.

11. All of the following are mild overdose reactions EXCEPT:
    a. Confusion
    b. Lightheadedness
    c. CNS depression
    d. Elevated heart rate

12. All of the following are epinephrine overdose reactions EXCEPT:
    a. Tremors
    b. Drop in blood pressure
    c. Perspiration
    d. Headache

13. All of the following are signs of an allergic reaction EXCEPT:
    a. Urticaria
    b. Pruritis
    c. Wheezing
    d. Bradycardia

CASE STUDY: MR. HALL

Mr. Hall requires periodontal scaling and root debriding. He has moderate periodontal disease and will require local anesthesia for comfort.

1. What topical anesthetic will you use?
2. What is your local anesthetic of choice?
3. List the nerves anesthetized for maxillary right quadrant.
4. What areas will be anesthetized?
5. What needle gauge should you use?
6. If you are right handed, what will be operator chair position?
7. What is the needle penetration site?
8. What are your landmarks?
9. How should the syringe be oriented?
10. Where will your hand rest?
11. What angle will you deposit the anesthesia?
12. What will your needle penetration depth be?
13. Describe your aspiration technique.
14. How much anesthetic will you deposit at first?
15. How long should it take you to deposit your initial anesthetic?

Age	48	SCENARIO
Gender	M	**EOE/IOE:**
Height	5'10"	Heavy supra- and subgingival calculus
Weight	160 lb	
B/P	150/55 mm Hg	**Periodontal Findings:**
Chief Complaint	Last dental exam was 8 years ago	4-6 mm generalized
		Radiographic Findings:
Medical History Current Medications	Seasonal allergies Claritin	Generalized moderate horizontal bone loss
Social History	Smokes 1 pack of cigarettes daily Drinks 3 beers a day	**Dental Findings:**

Performance Objective

By following a routine procedure that meets the stated protocols, the student will demonstrate the appropriate technique for **43-1 Oraqix Topical Anesthetic Application for Use During Scaling and Root Planing**

Evaluation and Grading Criteria

Instructor will assign grades for each performance criteria.

<u>3</u> Student competently met stated criteria
<u>2</u> Student required minimal assistance to meet criteria
<u>1</u> Student showed uncertainty when attempting criteria
<u>0</u> Student was not prepared and needs to repeat criteria
<u>N/A</u> Student was not evaluated

Performance Standards

Instructor shall identify steps that are critical with an asterisk (*)

Performance Criteria	*	Self	Peer	Instructor	Comments
EQUIPMENT: ■ Personal protective equipment ■ 2.5% Lidocaine and 2.5% Prilocaine cartridge ■ Oraqix dispenser ■ Blunt tip applicator ■ Cotton pliers/hemostat ■ 2 × 2 gauze					
STEPS 1. Assemble armamentarium.					
2. Place blunt tip applicator into the tip of the Oraqix dispenser and turn it to lock in place.					
3. Press reset button on body of handle.					
4. Load the cartridge stopper, end-first, into the body of the handle and join the tip to the applicator body. Twist to lock it in place.					
5. Partially remove the blunt tip applicator cap in order to bend the tip into a shape to suit individual patient or clinician needs.					
6. Select 3-4 teeth, apply Oraqix gel by tracing the gingival margin, and wait 30 seconds.					
7. Then move the blunt tip applicator directly into the periodontal pocket and fill it with the Oraqix gel.					
8. Documentation					
9. Prevention of Disease Transmission	*				
ADDITIONAL COMMENTS					

Performance Objective

By following a routine procedure that meets the stated protocols, the student will demonstrate the appropriate technique for **43-2 Loading the Metallic or Plastic Cartridge-Type Syringe**

Evaluation and Grading Criteria

Instructor will assign grades for each performance criteria.

<u>3</u> Student competently met stated criteria
<u>2</u> Student required minimal assistance to meet criteria
<u>1</u> Student showed uncertainty when attempting criteria
<u>0</u> Student was not prepared and needs to repeat criteria
<u>N/A</u> Student was not evaluated

Performance Standards

Instructor shall identify steps that are critical with an asterisk (*)

Performance Criteria	*	Self	Peer	Instructor	Comments
EQUIPMENT: ■ Personal protective equipment ■ Syringe ■ Needle ■ Gauze ■ Anesthetic cartridge ■ Topical anesthetic ■ Cotton-tip applicator ■ Hemostat or cotton pliers					
STEPS 1. Assemble armamentarium.					
2. Remove the sterilized syringe from its container and inspect to ensure the harpoon is sharp and straight.					
3. Retract the piston.					
4. Insert the cartridge.					
5. Use the thumb as shown to engage the harpoon in the plunger with gentle finger pressure. Another technique is to grasp the thumb ring in the palm of the hand and simultaneously rotate the harpoon while applying gentle pressure to engage it.					
6. Although no longer recommended, some clinicians may engage the harpoon by using gentle pressure on the plunger, as shown, and use the other hand to cover the glass as a precautionary measure should the cartridge glass break.					
7. Remove the clear or white plastic protective shield that covers the syringe and cartridge end of the needle.					
8. Screw the colored plastic-hubbed needle onto the syringe while simultaneously pushing it into the metal needle adapter of the syringe.					

Continued

Performance Criteria	*	Self	Peer	Instructor	Comments
9. Direct the needle away from the body, keep the hand at the needle hub, and loosen the colored plastic protective cap from the needle. Use a one-handed technique with the dominant thumb and index finger to pinch the cap to remove it.					
10. Let the cap slide off the needle and onto a piece of sterile gauze if not using a recapping device.					
11. Expel a few drops of solution to test for proper flow, and recap the needle using a safe recapping devise.					
12. Hold the syringe with one hand and glide the needle into the colored plastic cap lying on the instrument tray. Never attempt to hold cap with other hand because this may lead to an accidental needle stick exposure.					
13. Tilt the syringe upward to allow the cap to slide down to the hub and cover the needle. If the cap starts to slip off the needle, do not attempt to stop it with the other hand. Instead, let the cap fall on the instrument tray and begin the process again.					
14. Prevention of Disease Transmission	*				
ADDITIONAL COMMENTS					

COMPETENCY CHAPTER 43 LOCAL ANESTHESIA

Performance Objective

By following a routine procedure that meets the stated protocols, the student will demonstrate the appropriate technique for **43-3 Unloading the Breach-Loading Metallic or Plastic Cartridge-Type Syringe**

Evaluation and Grading Criteria

Instructor will assign grades for each performance criteria.

<u>3</u> Student competently met stated criteria
<u>2</u> Student required minimal assistance to meet criteria
<u>1</u> Student showed uncertainty when attempting criteria
<u>0</u> Student was not prepared and needs to repeat criteria
<u>N/A</u> Student was not evaluated

Performance Standards

Instructor shall identify steps that are critical with an asterisk (*)

Performance Criteria	*	Self	Peer	Instructor	Comments
EQUIPMENT: ■ Personal protective equipment ■ Syringe ■ Needle ■ Gauze ■ Anesthetic cartridge ■ Topical anesthetic ■ Cotton-tip applicator ■ Hemostat or cotton pliers					
STEPS 1. Retract the piston and pull the cartridge away from the needle with your thumb and forefinger as you retract the piston, until the harpoon disengages from the plunger.					
2. Remove the cartridge from the syringe by inverting the syringe, permitting the cartridge to fall free.					
3. Carefully unscrew the recapped needle, being careful not to accidentally discard the metal needle adaptor.					
4. Place the needle in a sharps container that is rigid, puncture proof, and leak resistant.					
5. Prevention of Disease Transmission	*				
ADDITIONAL COMMENTS					

Performance Objective

By following a routine procedure that meets the stated protocols, the student will demonstrate the appropriate technique for **43-4 Basic Techniques for a Successful Injection**

Evaluation and Grading Criteria

Instructor will assign grades for each performance criteria.

 <u>3</u> Student competently met stated criteria
 <u>2</u> Student required minimal assistance to meet criteria
 <u>1</u> Student showed uncertainty when attempting criteria
 <u>0</u> Student was not prepared and needs to repeat criteria
<u>N/A</u> Student was not evaluated

Performance Standards

Instructor shall identify steps that are critical with an asterisk (*)

Performance Criteria	*	Self	Peer	Instructor	Comments
EQUIPMENT: ■ Personal protective equipment ■ Syringe ■ Needle ■ Gauze ■ Anesthetic cartridge ■ Topical anesthetic ■ Cotton-tip applicator ■ Hemostat or cotton pliers					
STEPS 1. Assess health history. Take vital signs.					
2. Confirm care plan.					
3. Check armamentarium.					
4. Load the syringe and determine the syringe window and needle bevel orientation. The window of the cartridge should face the clinician, and the bevel of the needle should face the bone.					
5. Expel a few drops of the anesthetic solution to determine if a free flow of solution exists.					
6. Position the patient in a supine position (head and heart parallel to the floor) with the feet elevated slightly.					
7. Communicate with the patient to place positive ideas in the patient's mind about the injection. Tell the patient about the reasons for topical anesthetic (e.g., "I am applying a topical anesthetic to the tissue so that the remainder of the procedure will be much more comfortable."). Do not use words with a negative connotation, such as *injection, shot, pain,* or *hurt.* Instead, use less threatening terms such as *administer the LA.*					

Continued

Performance Criteria	*	Self	Peer	Instructor	Comments
8. Visualize or palpate to locate the penetration site.					
9. Dry the needle penetration site with sterile gauze.					
10. Apply topical anesthetic to needle penetration site for 1 to 2 minutes.					
11. In the case of palatal injections, when placing topical anesthetic on the injection site, apply considerable pressure with the cotton swab for a minimum of 1 minute before the injection. Move the swab immediately adjacent to the penetration site, and maintain pressure at this site during the injection.					
12. After the topical anesthetic swab is removed from the tissue, dry the penetration site.					
13. Pick up the prepared LA syringe and establish a firm hand rest. Never place the arm holding the syringe directly on the patient's arm or shoulder.					
14. Make the tissue taut at the penetration site by retracting it (except on the palate) using sterile gauze, aiding both visibility and atraumatic needle insertion.					
15. Keep syringe and needle out of the patient's line of vision.					
16. Gently insert the needle into the mucosa until the bevel is completely under the tissue.					
17. Observe and communicate with the patient. Watch for any signs of discomfort or distress.					
18. Deposit a few drops of anesthetic solution, pause for 5 seconds, and then advance the needle a few millimeters. Repeat process as you slowly advance to the deposition site. Communicate with the patient by saying, "To make you more comfortable, I will slowly deposit a little anesthetic at a time. To help you relax, please breathe slowly."					
19. Aspirate on arrival at the deposition site by pulling the thumb ring back gently. Movement of only 1 or 2 mm is needed. Tip of needle must remain unmoved.					
20. For most injections, rotate barrel of the syringe about 45 degrees, and aspirate a second time to ensure that the needle is not located inside a blood vessel and abutting against the wall of the vessel, providing a false-negative aspiration. In highly vascular areas, a triple aspiration is recommended.					
21. If no blood appears (negative aspiration), slowly deposit the LA solution at a rate of 1 mL/min for approximately 2 minutes for a full cartridge.					

Performance Criteria	*	Self	Peer	Instructor	Comments
22. If blood appears in the cartridge (positive aspiration), slowly withdraw the needle and communicate with your patient. Replace the cartridge and the needle and proceed with the injection.					
23. Observe and communicate with the patient. Watch for any signs of discomfort or distress. Reassure the patient with statements such as "I am depositing the solution slowly so this procedure will be comfortable for you." Slowly withdraw the needle when the indicated amount of anesthetic has been deposited.					
24. Slowly withdraw the needle when the indicated amount of anesthetic has been deposited.					
25. Resheath the needle using a recapping device (preferred) or the scoop technique (Figure P2.9). Multiple injections require checking the needle for barbs and/or sharpness. Slide the needle across a sterile 2 × 2 gauze square. If the gauze is snagged, indicating a barb is present, discard the needle.					
26. Observe the patient.					
27. Rinse the patient's mouth.					
28. Massage the tissue over the injection site when indicated.					
29. After 2-3 minutes, use a probe or rounded back of an instrument to test for anesthesia by first touching an area that is **not** anesthetized and then, secondly, touch the area that is anesthetized. The patient should have little or no sensation in the anesthetized area.					
30. Reassure the patient that numbness, tingling, and a sense of swelling, or the tooth feeling different, are normal responses.					
31. Record the injection sites in the patient's chart and include: ■ Area anesthetized and specific injection(s) given ■ Type of anesthetic used and type of vasoconstrictor and its concentration (ratio) ■ Gauge and type of needle(s) used ■ Total amount of solution administered (in milligrams and/or total cartridges) ■ Time the drug was administered ■ Patient reaction ■ Follow up with postoperative instructions, both verbally and in writing					
32. Prevention of Disease Transmission	*				
ADDITIONAL COMMENTS					

44 Nitrous Oxide-Oxygen Sedation

COMPETENCIES

1. Determine whether administration of N_2O-O_2 sedation is appropriate, based on the indications and contraindications for its use.
2. Provide information for patients about the advantages and disadvantages of N_2O-O_2 sedation for patient introduction to the procedure.
3. Recognize the signs and symptoms associated with safe and effective administration of N_2O-O_2 sedation.
4. Discuss equipment associated with N_2O-O_2 sedation, ensure patient and provider safety by monitoring the many safety features associated with N_2O-O_2 sedation equipment, and describe various delivery styles for sedation.
5. Describe administration and monitoring of N_2O-O_2 sedation, recognize potential complications that may occur during N_2O-O_2 sedation, and acknowledge appropriate response measures.

SHORT ANSWER QUESTIONS

1. List contraindications to using nitrous oxide sedation.

_____

_____

_____

_____

_____

_____

_____

_____

_____

2. List advantages of using N_2O-O_2 sedation.

_____

_____

_____

_____

_____

_____

_____

_____

_____

_____

_____

3. List disadvantages of using N_2O-O_2 sedation

_____

_____

_____

_____

_____

4. List normal signs of N_2O-O_2 sedation.

_____

_____

_____

_____

_____

_____

_____

_____

_____

_____

_____

5. What are the indications for using N_2O-O_2 sedation?

_____

_____

_____

_____

_____

_____

_____

_____

_____

FILL IN THE BLANK STATEMENTS

Select the best term from the chapter and complete the following statements.

1. _____ is the reduction of anxiety or agitation typically by administering sedative drugs.

2. _____ is a minimally depressed level of consciousness produced by a pharmacological method that retains the patient's ability to independently and continuously maintain an airway and respond *normally* to tactile stimulation and verbal command.

3. _____ is a drug-induced depression of consciousness during which patients respond *purposefully* to verbal commands, either alone or accompanied by light tactile stimulation.

4. _____ is a drug-induced depression of consciousness during which patients are not aroused easily, but they will respond to painful or repeated stimulation.

5. _____ is the administration of incremental doses of an intravenous or inhalation drug over time until a desired effect is reached.

6. _____ is difficulty breathing.

7. _____ is not breathing at all.

8. _____ is a procedure where a patient's cerebrospinal fluid is displaced with gas to better visualize the spine and/or brain.

9. _____ is the volume of gas inhaled and exhaled from a person's lungs per minute.

10. _____ is the measurement of a patient's carbon dioxide concentration over time.

MULTIPLE CHOICE QUESTIONS

Complete each question by circling the best answer.

1. A medical consult is recommended before N_2O-O_2 sedation is administered if a patient is taking bleomycin sulfate. Patients who are prescribed bleomycin sulfate should not be given 100% oxygen.
   a. Both statements are true.
   b. Both statements are false.
   c. The first statement is true and the second statement is false.
   d. The first statement is false and the second statement is true.

2. This sign is observed as the half-closed appearance of the eyelids or a slow blink rate.
   a. Verill's sign
   b. Psychosis
   c. Paranoid behavior
   d. Bell's palsy

3. Patients who have cardiovascular disease or hypertension are not candidates for N_2O-O_2 use. Nitrous oxide relaxes the heart vessels and helps decrease the stress on the heart.
   a. Both statements are true.
   b. Both statements are false.
   c. The first statement is true and the second statement is false.
   d. The first statement is false and the second statement is true.

4. The amount of nitrous oxide required for sedation is standard for all adult patients. The patient's prevailing mood prior to receiving nitrous oxide sedation may influence the depth of sedation.
   a. Both statements are true.
   b. Both statements are false.
   c. The first statement is true and the second statement is false.
   d. The first statement is false and the second statement is true.

5. Recommended minimum post-op time of 100% oxygen saturation is:
   a. 1 minute
   b. 5 minutes
   c. 10 minutes
   d. 15 minutes

6. All of the following are subjective symptoms of nitrous oxide sedation EXCEPT:
   a. Decreased pain memory
   b. Decreased awareness of time passing
   c. Feeling cold
   d. Arms and legs feeling heavy

7. All of the following are objective signs of desired level of nitrous oxide sedation EXCEPT:
   a. Ability to answer questions
   b. Normal eye reaction
   c. Normal blood pressure
   d. Decreased pulse

8. Contraindications to nitrous oxide use includes all of the following EXCEPT:
   a. Pregnancy
   b. COPD
   c. Fear of sedation
   d. Asthma

9. To reduce trace amounts of N_2O, the clinician should utilize a scavenging mask system and regularly check mask for leaks. The effects of chronic exposure to trace amounts of O_2 may include spontaneous abortion or birth defects.
   a. Both statements are true.
   b. Both statements are false.
   c. The first statement is true and the second statement is false.
   d. The first statement is false and the second statement is true.

10. Nitrous oxide and oxygen in amounts of 60% or less is considered minimal sedation. Combining nitrous oxide and another sedative is considered moderate sedation.
    a. Both statements are true.
    b. Both statements are false.
    c. The first statement is true and the second statement is false.
    d. The first statement is false and the second statement is true.

11. The administration of sedative medications to reduce anxiety is:
    a. General anesthesia
    b. Sedation
    c. Local anesthesia
    d. Titration

12. Anterograde amnesia is the perception that time:
    a. Passes quickly
    b. Passes slowly
    c. Stops
    d. Continues normally

13. The use of a scavenger system in the nitrous oxide delivery system is:
    a. Convenient
    b. Recommended
    c. Required
    d. Not necessary

CASE STUDY: MR. HAYES

Mr. Hayes is a 58-year-old male who is a patient of record in your office; however, he is sporadic in continued care. He was last seen by you 4 years ago when you informed him of his severe periodontal disease and need for periodontal therapy. He admitted to not taking care of his teeth and having an extreme fear of the dentist. He shared with you his personal story concerning the cause of his fear: He served in the military during Operation Desert Storm and was a prisoner of war. One of the methods his captors abused him was to connect a car battery to his mouth/teeth. He stated that it is now extremely stressful to have someone enter his mouth.

1. How can you help Mr. Hayes overcome his fear and provide him the oral health care he needs? Is nitrous oxide sedation a choice for him?
2. Would a consultation with an interprofessional team be warranted? What healthcare members would be appropriate?

Performance Objective

By following a routine procedure that meets the stated protocols, the student will demonstrate the appropriate technique for **44-1 Administration and Monitoring of Nitrous Oxide-Oxygen Sedation**

Evaluation and Grading Criteria

Instructor will assign grades for each performance criteria.

3 Student competently met stated criteria
2 Student required minimal assistance to meet criteria
1 Student showed uncertainty when attempting criteria
0 Student was not prepared and needs to repeat criteria
N/A Student was not evaluated

Performance Standards

Instructor shall identify steps that are critical with an asterisk (*)

Performance Criteria	*	Self	Peer	Instructor	Comments
1. Open tanks and turn on vacuum line. Check connections and equipment.					
2. Review patient's health history for any contraindications.					
3. Discuss risks/benefits/complications. Obtain consent.					
4. Obtain vital signs. Record them.					
5. Select hood and attach to hoses.					

6. Initiate flow of 100% oxygen.
  a. Adults initially at ~6 lpm; children initially at ~4 lpm
  b. Place nasal hood securely on patient. Gauze under the hood on the bridge of the nose may need to be placed.					

7. Determine minute volume. Fill the reservoir bag 2/3 full with oxygen by pressing the flush button.
  a. Decrease the flow if the bag fills.
  b. Increase the flow if it empties.					

8. Begin nitrous oxide administration with 10-20%. Maintain the established minute volume.					
9. Add N_2O in 5-10% increments and wait a few minutes for effect.					
10. Accomplish dental procedures when appropriate sedation is achieved.					
11. Terminate the N2O flow and correct the minute volume with 100% oxygen.					
12. Sit the patient up at least half way; leave the patient on oxygen for at least five minutes.					

Continued

Performance Criteria	*	Self	Peer	Instructor	Comments
13. Reassess emotional and physical state compared to when the patient was seated. Make sure the patient is alert and oriented.					
14. Check the vital signs. Record them. Ensure readings are similar to preoperative values.	.				
15. Dismiss the patient.					
16. Record the data: a. Pre- and post-vital signs b. Time sedation began and ended. c. Maximum concentration of nitrous oxide delivered and oxygenation time. d. Complications, if any, and corrective actions taken.					
17. Discard the disposables; clean, disinfect, and/or sterilize other components.					
18. Prevention of Disease Transmission	*				
ADDITIONAL COMMENTS					

Children and Adolescents

COMPETENCIES

1. Recognize the need for interprofessional collaborative practice to meet the health and oral health needs of children.
2. Promote oral health literacy among non-clinical and clinical primary care team members and caregivers.
3. Advocate for a healthy oral life span among children and adolescents.
4. Discuss fluoride consumption and therapy, including water fluoridation and fluoride toxicity.
5. Employ the Decayed, Missing, Filled Teeth (DMFT) and Decayed, Missing, Filled Surfaces (DMFS) indices to quantify clinical observations in children and adolescents.
6. Appreciate behavioral management strategies for pediatric patients during a dental care visit.

SHORT ANSWER QUESTIONS

1. To reduce the risk of caries in children, list the fluorides and percentages recommended by the American Dental Association.

_____

_____

_____

_____

_____

_____

2. List all items that should be included in a child's clinical dental record?

_____

_____

_____

_____

_____

_____

_____

_____

_____

_____

3. List caregiver tips for oral care in infants age birth to 1 year.

_____

_____

_____

_____

_____

_____

_____

_____

_____

_____

_____

_____

_____

4. List oral health challenges found in adolescents.

_____

_____

_____

_____

_____

_____

_____

_____

_____

_____

_____

FILL IN THE BLANK STATEMENTS

Select the best term from the chapter and complete the following statements.

1. _____ occurs when one or professionals from different disciplines work to ensure patient-centered care.

2. _____ is the degree to which individuals can obtain, process, and understand the basic health information and services need to make appropriate health decisions.

3. _____ is the presence of one or more decayed, missing, or filled primary teeth.

4. _____ can occur if recommended doses for fluoride additives are not followed.

5. _____ can occur if high levels of fluoride are ingested over long periods of time.

MULTIPLE CHOICE QUESTIONS

Complete each question by circling the best answer.

1. Breastfeeding after 1 year is a non-nutritive habit. Finger sucking is a non-nutritive habit.
   a. Both statements are true.
   b. Both statements are false.
   c. The first statement is true and the second statement is false.
   d. The first statement is false and the second statement is true.

2. DMFT scores for a typical adult is 0-32. Typical child dmft score is 0-20.
   a. Both statements are true.
   b. Both statements are false.
   c. The first statement is true and the second statement is false.
   d. The first statement is false and the second statement is true.

3. All of the following are included within the primary dentition EXCEPT:
   a. Incisors
   b. Canines
   c. Premolars
   d. Second molars

4. Vertical transmission of caries-causing bacteria occurs when saliva is passed from mother-child. Horizontal transmission of caries-causing bacteria is indirect exposure through eating utensils.
   a. Both statements are true.
   b. Both statements are false.
   c. The first statement is true and the second statement is false.
   d. The first statement is false and the second statement is true.

5. There is a higher incidence of accidents and trauma in children aged:
   a. birth-23 months
   b. 24-36 months
   c. 3-4 years
   d. 5-7 years

6. Which are typically the first primary teeth to exfoliate?
   a. Maxillary central incisors
   b. Mandibular central incisors
   c. Maxillary first molars
   d. Mandibular first molars

7. The best choice in choosing a protective mouth guard is:
   a. Custom fit
   b. In-office boil and bite
   c. In-home boil and bite
   d. Age-rated fit

8. A sum score would be used by a clinician measuring DMFT or DMFS in which of the following situations?
   a. Individual
   b. Population
   c. Sample
   d. Average

9. The most common symptom of acute fluoride toxicity is:
   a. Fluorosis
   b. GI upset
   c. Skeletal defects
   d. Anxiety

10. Dietary supplements of fluoride may be prescribed by a pediatrician or dentist. Dietary supplements of fluoride are available over-the-counter in small doses.
    a. Both statements are true.
    b. Both statements are false.
    c. The first statement is true and the second statement is false.
    d. The first statement is false and the second statement is true.

11. Infants older than 6 months should receive daily supplemental fluoride in liquid form. Children and adolescents should receive daily supplemental fluoride in liquid form or chewable tablets.
    a. Both statements are true.
    b. Both statements are false.
    c. The first statement is true and the second statement is false.
    d. The first statement is false and the second statement is true.

12. Mouthguards purchased for at-home fitting meet the standards recommended by the Academy of Sports Medicine. Appliances should be professionally fit and worn during all contact sports.
    a. Both statements are true.
    b. Both statements are false.
    c. The first statement is true and the second statement is false.
    d. The first statement is false and the second statement is true.

13. Which primary teeth are MOST susceptible to dental caries?
    a. Mandibular anterior
    b. Mandibular posterior
    c. Maxillary anterior
    d. Maxillary posterior

14. The Centers for Disease Control recommends an optimal fluoride concentration 1.0 mg/L to be added to municipal water systems. Fluoride occurs naturally in the earth and is found in soil, rocks, air, and water.
    a. Both statements are true.
    b. Both statements are false.
    c. The first statement is true and the second statement is false.
    d. The first statement is false and the second statement is true.

15. Establishing a dental home for children is recommended no later than:
    a. 3 months
    b. 6 months
    c. 1 year
    d. 2 years

16. One of the bacteria associated with periodontal disease during puberty and menses stages is:
    a. *Tannerella forsythensis*
    b. *Candida albicans*
    c. *Streptococcus mutans*
    d. Lactobacillus spp

CASE STUDY: SEBASTIAN

Sebastian is a 4-year-old active boy. He states his mouth hurts all the time. His mother was referred by his pediatrician to have a complete dental exam. Sebastian presents with rampant decay throughout his primary dentition. All anterior teeth are decayed to the gum line. He has abscesses on tooth #B and #I. Sebastian is covered under Medicaid insurance. The state mandates that all children who have Medicaid health insurance coverage also have a yearly dental exam and subsequent needed dental treatment or the parent loses benefits. The mother, a recovering drug addict, states that Sebastian drinks out of a sippy cup all day. She mostly gives him soda because he won't drink anything else. She admits that she serves Sebastian a lot of fast food and candy. He also throws frequent temper tantrums. After discussing his case with the pediatric dentist, a treatment plan included extracting all of Sebastian's infected teeth in a hospital setting. This will leave Sebastian with only a few natural posterior teeth. The pediatric dentist will attempt to place a pedo denture for Sebastian's anterior teeth.

1. What guidance do you provide the mother at this time?
2. What information do you give her for post-op OHI?
3. Develop a dental hygiene care plan for Sebastian and his mother following his surgery.

Using the data from this patient, develop a Human Needs Conceptual model for treatment.

Dental Hygiene Diagnosis (unmet human need)	Etiology (due to…)	Signs and Symptoms (evidenced by…)	Patient Goals (expected outcomes)
Protection from Health Risks			
Freedom from Fear and Stress			
Freedom from Pain			
Wholesome Facial Image			
Skin and Mucous Membrane Integrity of the Head and Neck			
Biologically Sound and Functional Dentition			
Conceptualization and Problem Solving			
Responsibility for Oral Health			

Performance Objective

By following a routine procedure that meets the stated protocols, the student will demonstrate the appropriate technique for **Professionally Applied Topical Fluoride Using the Tray Technique for In-Office Fluoride Treatment (Gel or Foam)**

Evaluation and Grading Criteria

Instructor will assign grades for each performance criteria.

<u>3</u> Student competently met stated criteria
<u>2</u> Student required minimal assistance to meet criteria
<u>1</u> Student showed uncertainty when attempting criteria
<u>0</u> Student was not prepared and needs to repeat criteria
<u>N/A</u> Student was not evaluated

Performance Standards

Instructor shall identify steps that are critical with an asterisk (*)

Performance Criteria	*	Self	Peer	Instructor	Comments
EQUIPMENT ■ Mouth mirror ■ Cotton forceps ■ Fluoride tray(s) ■ Cotton rolls ■ 1.23% acidulated phosphate fluoride (APF) or 2.0% sodium fluoride gel ■ Air syringe ■ Timer ■ Saliva ejector ■ 2 × 2 gauze ■ Tissues ■ 2-oz cup ■ Personal protective barriers and equipment barriers					
STEPS 1. Assemble equipment.					
2. Seat patient in upright position. Reiterate benefits and obtain informed consent.					
3. Try tray of appropriate size. Complete dentition must be covered, including areas of recession.					
4. Load fluoride gel into trays for maxillary and mandibular teeth: 2 mL maximum per tray for small children; 4 mL maximum per tray for large children (>44 lb), 2.5 mL maximum per tray for adults.					
5. Dry teeth with air syringe.					
6. Insert both trays in mouth.					
7. Press tray against teeth, and ask patient to close mouth and bite gently on trays or cotton rolls.					

Continued

Performance Criteria	*	Self	Peer	Instructor	Comments
8. Place saliva ejector over mandibular tray. Set timer for 4 minutes. Never leave patient unattended during procedure.					
9. Tilt chin down to remove trays.					
10. Ask patient to expectorate; suction excess fluoride from the mouth with saliva ejector.					
11. Instruct patient not to eat, drink, or rinse for 30 minutes.					
12. Record service in patient's chart under "services rendered"; e.g., "Applied topical APF fluoride gel to existing teeth for 4 minutes. Used stock trays to apply approx. 2 to 2.5 mL of 1.23% APF (insert brand name). Parent or caregiver consented to procedure; no complications or adverse reactions during treatment. Patient instructed not to eat or drink for 30 minutes."					
13. Prevention of Disease Transmission	*				
ADDITIONAL COMMENTS					

Performance Objective

By following a routine procedure that meets the stated protocols, the student will demonstrate the appropriate technique for **Professionally Applied Sodium Fluoride Varnish Using the Paint-On Technique**

Evaluation and Grading Criteria

Instructor will assign grades for each performance criteria.

3 Student competently met stated criteria
2 Student required minimal assistance to meet criteria
1 Student showed uncertainty when attempting criteria
0 Student was not prepared and needs to repeat criteria
N/A Student was not evaluated

Performance Standards

Instructor shall identify steps that are critical with an asterisk (*)

Performance Criteria	*	Self	Peer	Instructor	Comments
EQUIPMENT ■ Mouth mirror ■ 5% Sodium fluoride varnish (unit dosage) ■ Cotton-tip applicators or syringe applicator ■ Paper cup ■ Personal protective barriers and equipment barriers					
STEPS 1. Select unit dose fluoride varnish product; gather equipment and supplies for application.					
2. Provide patient with information about procedure; reiterate benefits. Obtain informed consent.					
3. Unless an oral prophylaxis has been performed at the same appointment, have patient cleanse teeth with toothbrush.					
4. Recline patient for ergonomic access to oral cavity.					
5. Wipe application area with gauze or cotton rolls and insert a saliva ejector. Can be applied in the presence of saliva and without a saliva ejector.					
6. Using a cotton-tip, brush, or applicator, apply 0.3 to 0.5 mL of varnish (unit dose) to clinical crown of teeth: application time is 1 to 3 minutes.					
7. Dental floss may be used to draw the varnish interproximally.					
8. Allow patient to rinse on completion of procedure.					
9. Remind patient to avoid eating hard foods, drinking hot or alcoholic beverages, brushing, and flossing until the next day or at least for 4 to 6 hours after application. Drink through a straw for the first few hours after application.					

Continued

Performance Criteria	*	Self	Peer	Instructor	Comments
10. Record service in patient's record under "Services Rendered," e.g., "Applied 0.3 mL of 5% (22,600 ppm) sodium fluoride varnish (insert brand name) per tooth. Patient consented to this procedure; no complications or adverse reactions during treatment. Patient instructed to keep varnish on the teeth for at least 4 to 6 hours or preferably until the next day. Patient told to drink through a straw and avoid hard foods, alcoholic and hot beverages, brushing, and flossing until preferably the next day to prolong the varnish treatment. Varnish can be removed the next day with toothbrushing and interdental cleaning."					
11. Prevention of Disease Transmission	*				
ADDITIONAL COMMENTS					

46 Pregnancy and Oral Health

1. Explain and classify the current state of evidence regarding maternal periodontal disease and adverse birth outcomes. Additionally, discuss potential oral manifestations during pregnancy.
2. Describe oral disease prevention and health behaviors during pregnancy, including professional oral healthcare during pregnancy and the prevention of ECC for infants.
3. Discuss the impact of low health literacy on the oral health of pregnant women and infants.
4. Describe healthcare provider guidelines on oral healthcare during pregnancy, including national priorities.
5. Collaborate interprofessionally with non–dental providers in fostering the importance of oral health for pregnant women.
6. Discuss various community programs that serve pregnant women.

SHORT ANSWER QUESTIONS

1. Childhood obesity may be the result of what adverse pregnancy condition?

_____

_____

2. List antibiotics women should avoid during pregnancy.

_____

_____

_____

_____

_____

3. List barriers to care for low-income pregnant women.

_____

_____

_____

_____

_____

_____

_____

_____

_____

_____

4. Describe strategies for positioning pregnant women in the dental chair.

_____

_____

_____

_____

_____

_____

_____

5. List strategies to help decrease incidence of early childhood caries.

_____

_____

_____

_____

_____

_____

_____

_____

_____

6. What are the Healthy People 2030 oral health objectives?

_____

_____

_____

_____

_____

_____

_____

_____

FILL IN THE BLANK STATEMENTS

Select the best term from the chapter and complete the following statements.

1. Another term for pregnancy is _____.

2. Together with their prenatal providers, _____ by the dental hygienist is recommended to pregnant women for educational information about balanced diet and dietary recommendations.

3. Poorly controlled diabetes in the first trimester of gestation can lead to _____.

4. _____ is an atypically large baby as a result of gestational diabetes.

5. _____ is an independent panel of experts in prevention and evidence-based medicine/dentistry that works to improve the health of all Americans.

6. _____ is a national initiative that sets and tracks health goals and objectives for Americans.

MULTIPLE CHOICE QUESTIONS

Complete each question by circling the best answer.

1. Mutans Streptococcus can be transmitted vertically from primary caregiver to child through saliva. Mutans Streptococcus can be transmitted horizontally from child to child.
   a. Both statements are true.
   b. Both statements are false.
   c. The first statement is true, the second statement is false.
   d. The first statement is false, the second statement is true.

2. There is moderately strong evidence that shows pregnant women who receive periodontal therapy reduce premature births (delivery before 37 weeks). There is modest research showing cause and effect between pregnant women with active periodontal disease and premature births.
   a. Both statements are true.
   b. Both statements are false.
   c. The first statement is true, the second statement is false.
   d. The first statement is false, the second statement is true.

3. Research demonstrates pregnant women:
   a. Who receive periodontal therapy reduce their chances of delivering pre-term births
   b. Who receive periodontal therapy are less likely to have baby birth weight less than 5.5 pounds
   c. Should only seek needed periodontal therapy after giving birth
   d. Should receive periodontal therapy only after the first trimester

4. Optimum levels of fluoride in municipal water systems to prevent caries is:
   a. .05 ppm
   b. 0.7 ppm
   c. 1.0 ppm
   d. 1.2 ppm

5. Consuming tap water over bottled water is preferred to aid in preventing caries. Commercial water filters remove essential fluoride ions from tap water.
   a. Both statements are true.
   b. Both statements are false.
   c. The first statement is true, the second statement is false.
   d. The first statement is false, the second statement is true.

6. Pregnancy gingivitis is caused by all of the following EXCEPT:
   a. Hormone fluctuations
   b. Substandard brushing
   c. Little or no interdental biofilm removal
   d. Lack of fluoridated water

7. Typical development of gestational diabetes in non-diabetic women manifests at:
   a. Conception
   b. 12 weeks
   c. 24 weeks
   d. 36 weeks

8. All of the following are subheadings of labels for prescription, over-the-counter, and supplemental medications EXCEPT:
   a. Adverse Pregnancy Outcomes
   b. Data
   c. Risk Summary
   d. Clinical Considerations

9. A vascular hyperplastic oral lesion that can manifest during pregnancy is:
   a. HPV
   b. Pemphigus vulgaris
   c. Hemangioma
   d. Pyogenic granuloma

10. Microbial shift from aerobic to anaerobic bacteria during pregnancy may manifest as:
    a. Localized periodontal bone loss
    b. Severe gingivitis
    c. Reversible tooth mobility
    d. NUG

11. An increase in carbohydrate consumption may contribute to increased caries incidence in pregnancy. An increase in oral hygiene practices may contribute to decreased caries incidence in pregnant women.
    a. Both statements are true.
    b. Both statements are false.
    c. The first statement is true, the second statement is false.
    d. The first statement is false, the second statement is true.

12. Thirty percent nitrous oxide may be used during pregnancy. Local anesthetics with epinephrine should not be used during pregnancy.
    a. Both statements are true.
    b. Both statements are false.
    c. The first statement is true, the second statement is false.
    d. The first statement is false, the second statement is true.

13. All of the following are safe to use during pregnancy EXCEPT:
    a. Chlorhexidine mouth rinse
    b. Lidocaine
    c. Tetracycline
    d. Nitrous oxide

14. All of the following should be avoided during pregnancy EXCEPT:
    a. Acetaminophen
    b. Moxifloxacin
    c. Clindamycin
    d. Ciprofloxacin

CASE STUDY: MS. BUENO

Age	20	SCENARIO
Gender	female	
Height	5'7"	**EOE/IOE:** Pyogenic granuloma 5 mm present facial to #6-7
Weight	130 lb	
B/P	130/80 mm Hg	**Periodontal Findings:** Generalized moderate inflammation Moderate subgingival calculus Moderate generalized BOP Probe depths 4-5 mm post
Chief Complaint	Gums are inflamed and sore Pain upper left third molar	
Medical History	5 months pregnant	**Radiographic Findings:** Slight bone loss posterior
Current Medications	none	**Dental Findings:** #3 carious lesion #14 carious lesion #30 carious lesion #32 is partially erupted and has an operculum #16 is fully erupted and symptomatic
Social History	Tobacco smoker ½ pack a day Marijuana smoker daily Occasional cocaine use	

Using the data from this patient, develop a Human Needs Conceptual model for treatment.

Dental Hygiene Diagnosis (unmet human need)	Etiology (due to…)	Signs and Symptoms (evidenced by…)	Patient Goals (expected outcomes)
Protection from Health Risks			
Freedom from Fear and Stress			
Freedom from Pain			
Wholesome Facial Image			
Skin and Mucous Membrane Integrity of the Head and Neck			
Biologically Sound and Functional Dentition			
Conceptualization and Problem Solving			
Responsibility for Oral Health			

1. Develop a detailed dental hygiene care plan for Ms. Bueno.
2. What educational information will you share with this patient?
3. What interprofessional interventions can you recommend?

_____

_____

_____

_____

_____

_____

_____

_____

_____

_____

_____

47 The Older Adult

COMPETENCIES

1. Explain and apply demographic characteristics of the aging population, including oral health disparities, to gain an increased understanding of best practices in customizing dental hygiene care for the older adult.
2. Define "geriatrics," discuss healthcare for older adults, and provide the rationale for performing a health assessment of an older person that includes a functional appraisal in addition to a review of health, dental, and personal histories.
3. Describe how health promotion, including the *Healthy People 2030* initiatives, contributes to an increase in the overall well-being and health, including oral health of older adults.
4. Describe and apply various theories of aging to the dental hygiene process of care.
5. Differentiate age-related health changes from those health and oral health conditions that occur as a result of acute or chronic diseases or medications in the elderly.
6. Customize each step in the process of dental hygiene care for elderly patients in light of their complex medical, dental, and related psychosocial issues.
7. Discuss the public health role of the dental hygienist in treating older adults in both the community-based and institutional setting.

SHORT ANSWER QUESTIONS

1. List and briefly describe the categories of aging.

_____

_____

_____

_____

_____

_____

2. List activities that are considered minimum to independent living for activities of daily living.

_____

_____

_____

_____

_____

_____

_____

_____

_____

3. List examples of instrumental activities of daily living that are more complex than ADL.

_____

_____

_____

_____

_____

4. List several caries prevention strategies for the older adult.

_____

_____

_____

_____

_____

_____

_____

_____

_____

_____

5. What are the causes of xerostomia in the older adult?

_____

_____

_____

_____

_____

_____

_____

_____

6. What are the negative effects of reduced salivary flow in the older adult?

_____

_____

_____

_____

_____

_____

_____

7. What are some common medications frequently used by the older adult?

_____

_____

_____

_____

_____

_____

_____

_____

8. Which subpopulation of older adult have the greatest oral needs and the most difficulty reaching dental services?

_____

_____

_____

_____

FILL IN THE BLANK STATEMENTS

Select the best term from the chapter and complete the following statements.

1. _____ is the average number of years that a person is expected to live.

2. The maximum length of life potentially possible is _____.

3. _____ is a medical specialty focusing on illnesses and treatments of old age.

4. _____ is the study of factors affecting normal aging process.

5. _____ is measured by calendar time since birth.

6. _____ is capability to maintain activity.

7. _____ are abilities fundamental to independent living.

8. _____ include complex activities to independent living.

9. _____ is the normal physiological aging process.

MULTIPLE CHOICE QUESTIONS

Complete each question by circling the best answer.

1. Which of the following has contributed to increased life expectancy?
   a. Increase in infant mortality
   b. Decrease in childhood obesity
   c. Increase in fertility rates
   d. Improved medical care

2. Stochastic theories view aging as random events that build over time. Non-stochastic theories view aging as a predetermined sequence through the life span.
   a. Both statements are true.
   b. Both statements are false.
   c. The first statement is true, the second statement is false.
   d. The first statement is false, the second statement is true.

3. There has been a dramatic decrease in edentulousness in older adults over the last 50 years. The decrease in edentulousness in older adults is contributed to better daily oral hygiene care.
   a. Both statements are true.
   b. Both statements are false.
   c. The first statement is true, the second statement is false.
   d. The first statement is false, the second statement is true.

4. Which of the following strategies will not contribute to preventing caries in older adults?
   a. Removable partial denture
   b. Saliva substitutes
   c. Professionally applied fluoride varnish
   d. Xylitol mints

5. The gradual deterioration of the immune system brought on by natural age advancement that involves both the host's capacity to respond to infections and the development of long-term immune memory is called:
   a. Innate immunity
   b. Adaptive immunity
   c. Immunosenescence
   d. Immunodeficiency

6. US Census data speculates that the number of older adults will continue to increase to 82.3 million in 2040. The number of older adults will grow to over 21% of the US population by 2040.
   a. Both statements are true.
   b. Both statements are false.
   c. The first statement is true, the second statement is false.
   d. The first statement is false, the second statement is true.

7. Older adults are more likely to smoke and drink alcohol than younger adults. Older adults are less likely to exercise regularly.
   a. Both statements are true.
   b. Both statements are false.
   c. The first statement is true, the second statement is false.
   d. The first statement is false, the second statement is true.

8. All of the following are age related tooth changes EXCEPT:
   a. Pulpal blood supply decreases
   b. Enamel becomes darker
   c. Dentinal sensitivity increases with recession
   d. Cementum has increased fluoride content

9. Older adults develop caries at a greater rate than younger adults. Root caries is least prevalent in older adults.
   a. Both statements are true.
   b. Both statements are false.
   c. The first statement is true, the second statement is false.
   d. The first statement is false, the second statement is true.

10. Which Human Needs Conceptual model deficits addresses chronic xerostomia and subsequent dry and inflamed oral mucosa?
    a. Protection from Health Risks
    b. Freedom from Pain
    c. Wholesome Facial Image
    d. Skin and Mucous Membrane Integrity of the Head and Neck

325

11. The term describing the normal process of growing old is:
    a. Aging
    b. Senescence
    c. Life span
    d. Existence

12. The following are oral tissue changes found in older adults EXCEPT:
    a. Thinning gingival epithelium
    b. Diminished keratinized tissue
    c. Increased gingival nerve degeneration
    d. Decrease in fibrous intercellular substance in the gingival connective tissue

CASE STUDY: MRS. WILSON

Age	85	SCENARIO
Gender	female	**EOE/IOE:** Xerostomia, dry painful tissues Generalized moderate to heavy biofilm Slight calculus generalized
Height	5'4"	
Weight	180 lb	
B/P	130/85 mm Hg	
Chief Complaint	Soreness in oral tissues	
Medical History	Knee replacement 5 years ago, no premed necessary per MD High blood pressure High cholesterol Type II diabetes HbA1c 6.8 Arthritis, particularly in hands/feet. Has trouble with dexterity. Slight hearing impaired – wears hearing aids	**Periodontal Findings:** 1-3 mm recession generalized Probe readings 1-3 mm Moderate BOP generalized **Radiographic Findings:** Generalized horizontal bone loss consistent with moderate periodontal disease diagnosis **Dental Findings:** Facial root caries on #6, #13 Demineralization on facial surfaces generalized
Current Medications	Lipitor Hydrochlorothiazide Norvasc Metformin Aleve prn	
Social History	Widowed 10 years Never smoked Social drinker, one glass of wine a month Lives alone, daughter and granddaughter live a few miles away and check on her daily Unsteady on her feet occasionally, requires some assistance when walking Has Medicare and supplemental dental insurance policy No longer able to drive, unable to attend church and social functions Receives Meals on Wheels during the week Patient reported feeling depressed that she cannot socialize very often. She also stated she does not want to be placed in a long term care facility	

1. What is your dental hygiene diagnosis for this patient?
2. Develop a care plan for Mrs. Wilson.
3. What interprofessional interventions that would benefit this patient?
   a. Primary Care Physician
   b. Physical Therapist
   c. Mental Health Professional
   d. Social Services
4. What patient education topics should be discussed? Who should also be involved with Mrs. Wilson's care?
5. What goals will you set for Mrs. Wilson?

_____

_____

_____

_____

_____

_____

_____

_____

_____

_____

_____

_____

_____

_____

Using the data from this patient, develop a Human Needs Conceptual model for treatment.

Dental Hygiene Diagnosis (unmet human need)	Etiology (due to...)	Signs and Symptoms (evidenced by...)	Patient Goals (expected outcomes)
Protection from Health Risks			
Freedom from Fear and Stress			
Freedom from Pain			
Wholesome Facial Image			
Skin and Mucous Membrane Integrity of the Head and Neck			
Biologically Sound and Functional Dentition			
Conceptualization and Problem Solving			
Responsibility for Oral Health			

48 Cardiovascular Disease

COMPETENCIES

1. Apply knowledge of cardiovascular disease and its risk factors while critically evaluating the relationship between cardiovascular diseases and periodontal disease.
2. Distinguish the etiology, risk factors, signs, symptoms, and medical and dental hygiene care of patients with hypertensive cardiovascular disease, history of angina or myocardial infarction, coronary heart disease, congestive heart failure, congenital heart disease, valvular heart defects, and rheumatic heart disease.
3. Identify the types of cardiovascular surgery and their implications for dental hygiene treatment.
4. Discuss oral manifestations of cardiovascular medications.
5. Understand implications in developing a dental hygiene diagnosis and care plan for a patient with cardiovascular disease, including comprehensive preventive and therapeutic dental hygiene services as well as the management of cardiac emergencies.

SHORT ANSWER QUESTIONS

1. Give examples of non-modifiable risk factors for cardiovascular disease.

_____

_____

_____

_____

_____

_____

_____

2. What stage of hypertension is the blood pressure reading at or above 130-139 mm Hg systolic or 80-89 mm Hg diastolic?

_____

3. List the emergency steps to be taken by the dental hygienist if a patient presents with third-degree heart block.

_____

_____

_____

_____

_____

4. Give examples of modifiable risk factors for cardiovascular disease.

_____

_____

_____

_____

_____

_____

_____

_____

_____

5. What is the most common valvular heart defect?

_____

6. What are commonly prescribed anticoagulants that may have the oral implication of increased bleeding?

_____

_____

_____

_____

_____

_____

_____

FILL IN THE BLANK STATEMENTS

Select the best term from the chapter and complete the following statements.

1. _____ is known as an abnormality of the heart's structure and function caused by deviant heart development before birth.

2. _____ is a condition characterized by myocardial dysfunction that leads to diminished cardiac output or abnormal circulatory congestion.

3. A _____ is caused by the blocking of electrical impulses that control the heart, from the atria to the ventricles at the AV node.

4. _____ is slowness of the heartbeat as evidenced by pulse rate of less than 60 beats per minute.

5. _____ is also known as a heart attack.

6. A _____ is an irregularity of a heartbeat caused by an auditory turbulent flow of blood through a valve that has failed to close.

MULTIPLE CHOICE QUESTIONS

Complete each question by circling the best answer.

1. Research indicates that the immune response to periodontal disease may increase cardiovascular risk. Essential idiopathic hypertension is the most common type of hypertension.
   a. Both statements are true.
   b. Both statements are false.
   c. The first statement is true and the second statement is false.
   d. The first statement is false and the second statement is true.

2. All of the following medical conditions may increase the risk of a medical emergency due to stress and fear EXCEPT:
   a. Hypertension
   b. Mitral valve prolapse
   c. Previous myocardial infarction
   d. Angina pectoris

3. Patients who have had heart transplants are at a risk for infection and organ rejection. A consultation with the patient's cardiologist is necessary if invasive dental services are to be performed within 6 months of the transplant.
   a. Both statements are true.
   b. Both statements are false.
   c. The first statement is true and the second statement is false.
   d. The first statement is false and the second statement is true.

4. Patients who have right-sided heart failure have decreased oxygenated blood coming from the lungs, resulting in increased fluid and blood in the lungs, causing dyspnea on exertion, shortness of breath on lying supine, cough, and sleep. Patients who have left-sided heart failure have blood return from the body, resulting in systemic venous congestion and peripheral edema.
   a. Both statements are true.
   b. Both statements are false.
   c. The first statement is true and the second statement is false.
   d. The first statement is false and the second statement is true.

5. All of the following are common congenital heart malformations EXCEPT:
   a. Ventricular septal defect
   b. Atrial septal defect
   c. Angina pectoris
   d. Patent ductus arteriosus

6. All of the following are non-modifiable risk factors for hypertension EXCEPT:
   a. Race
   b. Age
   c. Diet
   d. Genetics

7. All of the following conditions require antibiotic premedication prior to dental treatment to prevent infective endocarditis EXCEPT:
   a. Repaired CHD with residual defects at the site
   b. Mitral valve prolapse
   c. Previous infective endocarditis
   d. Unrepaired cyanotic congenital heart disease (CHD)

8. All of the following are considered valvular defects EXCEPT:
   a. Mitral valve
   b. Aortic valve
   c. Bicuspid valve
   d. Tricuspid valve

9. Which calcium channel blocker has oral implications of decreased salivary flow and gingival enlargement?
   a. Cardizem
   b. Calciparine
   c. Nitroglycerine
   d. Coumadin

10. Which ACE inhibitor has oral implication of xerostomia, taste alteration, and oral ulcerations?
    a. Lisinopril
    b. Benazepril
    c. Enalapril
    d. Captopril

11. Narrowing of the lumen of coronary arteries occurs when there are deposition of fibro-fatty substances containing lipids and cholesterol. Deposits of fibro-fatty substances thicken the lumen of coronary arteries and are eventually obstructed.
    a. Both statements are true.
    b. Both statements are false.
    c. The first statement is true and the second statement is false.
    d. The first statement is false and the second statement is true.

12. All of the following are alternative terms for a heart attack EXCEPT:
    a. Myocardial infarction
    b. Coronary thrombosis
    c. Coronary occlusion
    d. Ischemia

Mr. Manaheim reports having a very stressful home life. His oldest child is addicted to heroin and his youngest child is developmentally delayed. He works as a sales associate in a local car dealership. He reports that he has a lot of fear of dental visits. Complete the Human Needs Concept Model and develop a dental hygiene care plan for Mr. Mamahein.

Age	45	SCENARIO
Gender	male	**EOE/IOE:**
Height	6'1"	Coated tongue
Weight	250 lb	Nicotine stomatitis
B/P	170/110 mm Hg	Heavy biofilm generalized Heavy calculus generalized
Chief Complaint	10 years since last dental exam, bleeding gums	Heavy extrinsic brown stain generalized
Medical History Current Medications	High blood pressure Previous heart attack 3 months ago Concerned about the tobacco staining Lasix Cardizem Lopressor	**Periodontal Findings:** 5-6 mm pockets posterior, 3-4 mm pockets anterior, generalized 2-3 mm recession Gingival tissues erythematous, bulbous with spontaneous bleeding generalized Fistula present on the buccal of tooth #18 Class I furcation on all molars Class I mobility on # 24-25 **Radiographic Findings:** Perio/endo lesion #18 Caries #14 **Dental Findings:** Numerous carious lesions
Social History	Smokes one pack of cigarettes a day, smokes cigars 1-2 times a week Drinks 8 oz of whiskey a day Primary care physician recommended that patient have a dental exam	

1. Can he be seen today? Why or why not?
2. How would you address his fear?
3. Does he need premedication?

_____

_____

_____

_____

_____

_____

_____

_____

_____

_____

_____

Using the data from this patient, develop a Human Needs Conceptual model for treatment.

Dental Hygiene Diagnosis (unmet human need)	Etiology (due to…)	Signs and Symptoms (evidenced by…)	Patient Goals (expected outcomes)
Protection from Health Risks			
Freedom from Fear and Stress			
Freedom from Pain			
Wholesome Facial Image			
Skin and Mucous Membrane Integrity of the Head and Neck			
Biologically Sound and Functional Dentition			
Conceptualization and Problem Solving			
Responsibility for Oral Health			

49 Diabetes

COMPETENCIES

1. Differentiate between prediabetes, type 1 and type 2 diabetes, and gestational diabetes in terms of prevalence, characteristics, pathophysiology, and potential complications.
2. Discuss the two-way relationship between diabetes and periodontal disease. In addition, provide client education regarding self-monitoring, lifestyle changes, and pharmacological therapy to engage patients with diabetes as co-therapists in management of diabetes and oral care.
3. Plan dental hygiene care, including all steps in the process of care, for a person with diabetes and periodontal disease, and collaborate interprofessionally with a patient's primary healthcare provider.
4. Recognize a diabetic emergency and take appropriate action for management.
5. Assist patients at risk for diabetes in preventing diabetes and recommend referral for screening.

SHORT ANSWER QUESTIONS

1. List interventions that may prevent type 2 diabetes.

_____

_____

_____

_____

_____

_____

_____

_____

2. What are risks associated with developing type 2 diabetes?

_____

_____

_____

_____

_____

_____

_____

_____

_____

_____

_____

3. What are the four types of injectable insulin for patients with type 1 diabetes?

_____

_____

_____

_____

_____

_____

_____

_____

4. What are the long-term effects on overall health due to type 1 and type 2 diabetes?

_____

_____

_____

_____

_____

_____

_____

_____

5. Which blood test is used to monitor overall glycemic control?

_____

_____

_____

_____

6. List intraoral findings that may be present in patients with uncontrolled diabetes.

_____

_____

_____

_____

_____

_____

_____

7. Describe interventions to be used with a patient with controlled diabetes.

_____

_____

_____

_____

_____

_____

_____

_____

8. What medical emergencies might you encounter with a patient with diabetes?

_____

_____

_____

_____

_____

_____

_____

_____

_____

_____

9. What is the role of the dental hygienist when providing care to a patient with diabetes?

_____

_____

_____

_____

_____

_____

_____

_____

10. What are the warning signs of type 1 diabetes?

_____

_____

_____

_____

_____

_____

_____

_____

11. In addition to type 1 diabetes warning signs (question 10), what other signs of type 2 diabetes may be apparent?

_____

_____

_____

_____

_____

_____

_____

_____

_____

12. List the oral assessment findings common in patients with uncontrolled diabetes.

_____

_____

_____

_____

_____

_____

_____

_____

_____

_____

_____

FILL IN THE BLANK STATEMENTS

Select the best term from the chapter and complete the following statements.

1. _____ is a condition where there are high levels of blood glucose.

2. _____ is abnormal amounts of lipids in the blood.

3. _____ is damage to peripheral nerves often caused by diabetes.

4. _____ is a serious complication of diabetes that occurs when the body produces high levels of ketones.

5. _____ is a severe increase in urine volume.

6. _____ is excessive thirst.

7. _____ is extreme food consumption with no associated weight gain.

8. _____ is also known as burning mouth.

MULTIPLE CHOICE QUESTIONS

Complete each question by circling the best answer.

1. Type 1 diabetes is the most common form of diabetes. Type 2 diabetes is preventable.
   a. Both statements are true.
   b. Both statements are false.
   c. The first statement is true, the second statement is false.
   d. The first statement is false, the second statement is true.

2. Type 2 diabetes is often tied to genetics. Cardiovascular disease is the major contributor to developing type 2 diabetes.
   a. Both statements are true.
   b. Both statements are false.
   c. The first statement is true, the second statement is false.
   d. The first statement is false, the second statement is true.

3. Insulin is classified as what type of hormone?
   a. Catabolic
   b. Anabolic
   c. Steroid
   d. Analog

4. All of the following diseases have an increased incidence in patients with diabetes EXCEPT:
   a. Cerebrospinal
   b. Atherosclerotic
   c. Cardiovascular
   d. Cerebrovascular

5. What A1C levels indicate prediabetes?
   a. 4.0-5.8%
   b. 5.9-6.4%
   c. 6.5-7.9%
   d. 8.0+%

6. Normal blood glucose concentration is:
   a. 40-79 mg/dL
   b. 80 to 120 mg/dL
   c. 121 to 160 mg/dL
   d. 161 to 200 mg/dL

7. All patients with type 1 diabetes require antibiotic premedication. When using local anesthesia in patients with type 1 diabetes, use minimal epinephrine to avoid raising blood sugar.
   a. Both statements are true.
   b. Both statements are false.
   c. The first statement is true, the second statement is false.
   d. The first statement is false, the second statement is true.

8. A medical emergency whereby your patient with type 1 diabetes has a blood glucose concentration of <70 mg/dL is indicative of:
   a. Ketoacidosis
   b. Lactic acidosis
   c. Hypoglycemia
   d. Diabetic coma

9. Managing type 2 diabetes includes all of the following EXCEPT:
   a. Increased exercise
   b. Healthy diet
   c. Weight reduction
   d. Monitoring daily insulin injections

10. Long-term negative systemic effects from type 1 diabetes include kidney and eye diseases. Long-term negative systemic effects from type 2 diabetes includes atherosclerosis and hypertension.
    a. Both statements are true.
    b. Both statements are false.
    c. The first statement is true, the second statement is false.
    d. The first statement is false, the second statement is true.

11. Patients should only receive dental hygiene therapy if their blood glucose levels are:
    a. 40-69 mg/dL
    b. 70-200 mg/dL
    c. More than 200 mg/dL
    d. Any level is acceptable

12. Blood glucose levels that rise to more than 400 mg/dL is:
    a. Hyperglycemia
    b. Hypoglycemia
    c. Diabetic ketoacidosis
    d. Ketonemia

13. Keto acids and acetones that are produced as a result of catabolism of fatty acids is:
    a. Lipolysis
    b. Polydipsia
    c. Polyuria
    d. Hyperglycemia

14. A patient with diabetes and periodontal disease with a HbA1c level of greater than 7% would have a periontitis grade of:
    a. A
    b. B
    c. C
    d. D

CASE STUDY: MR. SWEENEY

Age	52	SCENARIO
Gender	male	**EOE/IOE:**
Height	5'11"	
Weight	180 lb	
B/P	138/85 mm Hg	**Periodontal Findings:**
Chief Complaint	Last dental cleaning was 2 years ago, "I have anxiety in the dental office"	Generalized moderate gingival inflammation Probe readings 4-5 mm posterior with 1-mm recession, 2-3 mm anterior with 2 mm recession
Medical History	Diabetes type 1 for 10 years insulin pump – 2 years	Moderate biofilm generalized Moderate calculus generalized
	24-hour blood sugar test results average 185 mL/dL	**Radiographic Findings:** #2 caries MO #18 caries MOD Generalized moderate horizontal bone loss
	3-month A1C level 8.2	
	Reports not eating healthy meals	**Dental Findings:** #2, #18 require restorations
Current Medications	Lispro, Glargine	
Social History	3-6 beers weekly No tobacco use	

Develop a detailed dental hygiene care plan for Mr. Sweeney.

1. What preparations will you make to address a possible medical emergency?
2. Is this patient controlled? Can he be treated in your office today?
3. Does he need premedication?
4. What topics will you cover during oral hygiene education?

_____

_____

_____

_____

_____

_____

_____

_____

_____

_____

_____

_____

_____

Using the data from this patient, develop a Human Needs Conceptual model for treatment.

Dental Hygiene Diagnosis (unmet human need)	Etiology (due to…)	Signs and Symptoms (evidenced by…)	Patient Goals (expected outcomes)
Protection from Health Risks			
Freedom from Fear and Stress			
Freedom from Pain			
Wholesome Facial Image			
Skin and Mucous Membrane Integrity of the Head and Neck			
Biologically Sound and Functional Dentition			
Conceptualization and Problem Solving			
Responsibility for Oral Health			

50 Cancer

COMPETENCIES

1. Explain the incidence of cancer and oral cancer, as well as the risk factors and common signs and symptoms.
2. Describe various forms of cancer therapy.
3. Discuss various oral complications from cancer treatment, including complications specific to chemotherapy, the rationale for bisphosphonate use, and the potential for osteonecrosis.
4. Explain the dental hygiene process of care for patients with cancer before, during, and after cancer therapy in collaboration with the interprofessional oncology team.

SHORT ANSWER QUESTIONS

1. List behaviors that may reduce the incidence of oral cancer.

_____

_____

_____

_____

_____

_____

_____

_____

2. List risk factors for oral cancer.

_____

_____

_____

_____

3. List oral complications associated with oral cancer treatment.

_____

_____

_____

_____

_____

4. Describe the recommended fluoride regimen for patients who will receive oral radiation.

_____

_____

_____

_____

5. What is the direct effect of radiation on tissues and bones?

_____

_____

_____

_____

6. What are the contents of a mucolytic cleansing solution?

_____

_____

_____

_____

_____

7. List common signs of oral cancer.

_____

_____

_____

_____

_____

_____

8. List potential ACUTE complications of head and neck radiation.

_____

_____

_____

_____

_____

_____
_____
_____
_____
_____

9. List potential CHRONIC complications of head and neck radiation.

_____
_____
_____
_____
_____
_____
_____

FILL IN THE BLANK STATEMENTS

Select the best term from the chapter and complete the following statements.

1. _____ is another term for cancer.

2. _____ is another term for cancer causing.

3. _____ is another term for likely outcome.

4. _____ relieves pain without directly treating the cause.

5. _____ occurs when plant alkaloid chemotherapeutic agents damage healthy nerve tissue.

6. _____ is the limited jaw range of opening or motion.

7. About one-third of oral cancers are related to _____.

MULTIPLE CHOICE QUESTIONS

Complete each question by circling the best answer.

1. What factors do not disproportionately affect cancer prevention, detection, and treatment?
   a. Geography
   b. Income
   c. Education
   d. Drug misuse

2. There has been an increase in oral cancer cases per year in Caucasians due to:
   a. HIV
   b. HPV
   c. Tobacco use
   d. Alcohol use

3. Approximately 9 out of 10 oral cancers are:
   a. Squamous cell carcinoma
   b. Basal cell carcinoma
   c. Malignant
   d. Detectible through head and neck exam

4. Which vaccine has been proven to reduce the risk of HPV?
   a. Gardasil 9
   b. MMR
   c. Small pox
   d. Hepatitis B

5. Which government agency recommends the HPV vaccine to teens and young adults?
   a. FDA
   b. ADA
   c. AMA
   d. CDC

6. The most common sites for oral cavity cancer are all of the following EXCEPT:
   a. Floor of the mouth
   b. Ventral surface of the tongue
   c. Lateral borders of the tongue
   d. Soft palate

7. Cancer therapy that uses the patient's own immune system to destroy cancer cells is:
   a. Targeted therapy
   b. Immunotherapy
   c. Hormone therapy
   d. Precision medicine

8. Mucositis is painful side effect of oral radiation therapy. Mucositis is a permanent side effect of oral radiation therapy.
   a. Both statements are true.
   b. Both statements are false.
   c. The first statement is true, the second statement is false.
   d. The first statement is false, the second statement is true.

9. Patients who are to receive bisphosphonate therapy should improve oral hygiene before medication regimen begins. Antibiotic prophylaxis is not recommended for patients who take bisphosphonates prior to invasive oral treatment.
   a. Both statements are true.
   b. Both statements are false.
   c. The first statement is true, the second statement is false.
   d. The first statement is false, the second statement is true.

10. A patient presents with mucositis during head and neck radiation. Which Human Needs Model deficit is the BEST choice?
    a. Freedom from Pain
    b. Wholesome Facial Image
    c. Skin and Mucous Membrane Integrity of the Head and Neck
    d. Biologically Sound and Functional Dentition

11. A patient presents with an oral infection related to chemotherapy-induced immunosuppression. All of the following care guidelines for dental hygiene treatment EXCEPT:
    a. The patient's absolute neutrophil count is >1000/mm^3
    b. Prescribe prophylactic antibiotics if the patient has a central venous catheter
    c. The patient may need extra time for periodontal therapy
    d. Encourage oral hydration with water, ices, and saliva substitutes

Lucas, your 35-year-old male patient, presented with a lesion on the facial mucosa on the left mandible that was recently diagnosed with squamous cell carcinoma. He is a smoker and drinks six beers a day. His preventive care appointments are sporadic. He was diagnosed with type II periodontal disease 1 year ago, and quadrant scaling was recommended. He also has several carious lesions. He states that fear of treatment has prevented him from completing his proposed dental plan.

Create a dental hygiene care plan listing specific professional treatment strategies and home care plan.

_____

_____

_____

_____

_____

_____

_____

_____

_____

_____

_____

_____

_____

_____

_____

_____

_____

_____

COMPETENCIES

1. Discuss the history of human immunodeficiency virus (HIV) in relation to the current status of HIV and AIDS.
2. Describe HIV modes of transmission, HIV latency and immune status, and pharmaceutical management for PWH.
3. Elucidate why people with weakened immune systems may be more vulnerable to an opportunistic infection (OI) and describe the epidemiology of HIV infection and AIDS.
4. Explain the concept of the HIV continuum.
5. Describe the dental hygiene process of care for PWH, including systemic health and oral health considerations.
6. Discuss the risk of HIV infection among healthcare workers and mechanisms to prevent transmission in the dental office.
7. Understand the National HIV/AIDS strategy inclusive of the plan to end the HIV epidemic in the U.S.

SHORT ANSWER QUESTIONS

1. What are the seven stages of HIV life cycle?

_____

_____

_____

_____

_____

_____

_____

2. List symptoms of an acute HIV infection.

_____

_____

_____

_____

_____

_____

_____

_____

_____

_____

3. List factors that contribute to racial disparities and HIV status.

_____

_____

_____

_____

_____

_____

4. What common fungal infections are found in patients with HIV?

_____

_____

_____

_____

_____

5. What are the characteristics and recommendations of patients who are prescribed HIV pre-exposure prophylaxis drug therapy?

_____

_____

_____

_____

_____

_____

_____

_____

_____

_____

FILL IN THE BLANK STATEMENTS

Select the best term from the chapter and complete the following statements.

1. _____ is an HIV virus particle containing a lipid-coated RNA core.

2. _____ is the white blood cell essential to cell-mediated immunity.

3. _____ is the ability of certain chemicals or mediator cells to destroy living cells.

4. _____ is also known as lymph node enlargement.

5. _____ is also known as a sore throat.

6. _____ is also known as aching muscles.

7. _____ is also known as aching joints.

Complete each question by circling the best answer.

1. The most successful pharmacological breakthrough to improve HIV prognosis was:
   a. Fusion inhibitors
   b. Viral protease
   c. Protease inhibitors
   d. CCR5 inhibitors

2. All of the following have contributed to the decrease in HIV infections EXCEPT:
   a. Pharmacology
   b. Universal precautions
   c. Education
   d. Prevention

3. HIV-2 is primarily found in:
   a. US
   b. Europe
   c. West Africa
   d. South America

4. All of the following are transmission routes for HIV infection EXCEPT:
   a. Contaminated needles
   b. Sexual contact
   c. Breast milk
   d. Saliva

5. Period of time during which specific antibodies develop and become detectible in a blood test is:
   a. Immune response
   b. Delta-32 mutation
   c. Seroconversion
   d. Adaptive immunity

6. Acute HIV infection is characterized by:
   a. CD4 count increase
   b. DNA conversion to RNA
   c. Seroconversion
   d. Primary viremia

7. Daily antiretroviral treatment for HIV includes all of the following EXCEPT:
   a. Improves quality of life
   b. Reduces the risk of transmission
   c. Reduces the concentration of the virus in circulation
   d. Eliminates the virus at the cellular level

8. Almost half of the population living with HIV is under age 50. CDC guidelines recommend HIV testing for everyone between the ages of 13 and 64.
   a. Both statements are true.
   b. Both statements are false.
   c. The first statement is true, the second statement is false.
   d. The first statement is false, the second statement is true.

9. Percent of the population who are unaware of their positive HIV status is:
   a. 10-13%
   b. 14-18%
   c. 19-25%
   d. 26-35%

10. Planning for oral health care for patients with HIV+ status is vastly different from the HIV negative counterparts. Using ultrasonic instrumentation is a contraindication for patients with HIV+ status.
    a. Both statements are true.
    b. Both statements are false.
    c. The first statement is true, the second statement is false.
    d. The first statement is false, the second statement is true.

11. The most common oral manifestation that occurs in patients who are HIV+ is:
    a. Herpetic lesions
    b. HPV
    c. NUP
    d. Oral candidiasis

12. The level of oral health care to be provided to patients with HIV is based on their blood-borne serostatus. Standard universal precautions are sufficient to protect healthcare workers when providing oral health care to patients with HIV+ status.
    a. Both statements are true.
    b. Both statements are false.
    c. The first statement is true, the second statement is false.
    d. The first statement is false, the second statement is true.

13. Comprehensive dental hygiene therapy for patients with HIV+ status should follow the same guidelines as patients who do not have HIV. Patients with HIV+ require more frequent dental hygiene visits than patients who do not have HIV.
    a. Both statements are true.
    b. Both statements are false.
    c. The first statement is true, the second statement is false.
    d. The first statement is false, the second statement is true.

14. HIV infection rates have slowly increased over the last 20 years. The most prevalent population affected with HIV is African American men.
    a. Both statements are true.
    b. Both statements are false.
    c. The first statement is true, the second statement is false.
    d. The first statement is false, the second statement is true.

15. How many days following exposure will acute HIV infection syndrome occur?
    a. 1 to 14
    b. 6 to 56
    c. 15 to 30
    d. 14 to 60

CASE STUDY: MR. JOHNSON

Age	30	SCENARIO
Gender	male	**EOE/IOE:**
Height	6'2"	Severe candidiasis present throughout his oral tissues, the palate and tongue
Weight	200 lb	
B/P	135/80 mm Hg	
Chief Complaint	Pain on tongue and roof of mouth	**Periodontal Findings:**
Medical History	HIV+ Depression CD4 T-lymphocyte count at 350 platelet count 20,000/mcl and neutrophils at 400 cells µL	Probe readings generalized 2-3 mm, slight BOP interproximal areas of posterior teeth, slight biofilm generalized, slight calculus generalized, moderate calculus mandibular anterior **Radiographic Findings:** Stable dentition
Current Medications	Zovirax Ativan Retrovir Crixivan Triazolam	**Dental Findings:** stable dentition
Social History	non-smoker non-drinker	

Develop a treatment plan for Mr. Johnson. What is his periodontal status? Do you need medical clearance to proceed with dental hygiene therapy? What educational topics would you cover with him? Can you treat him today?

_____

_____

_____

_____

_____

_____

_____

_____

_____

_____

_____

_____

_____

_____

52 Palliative Oral Care

COMPETENCIES

1. Discuss palliative care and explain palliative dental hygiene oral care.
2. Describe the role of the dental hygienist and appropriate palliative dental hygiene oral care practices in any setting.
3. Advocate for inclusion of dental hygienists as an essential healthcare provider in legislation across the healthcare system.
4. Apply the dental hygiene process of care to persons who are palliative and/or at the end of life.
5. Recognize the signs of aging, frailty, and oral complications manifested in the mouth during the process of dying and death.
6. Integrate strategies of palliative dental hygiene oral care used to accommodate increasing oral frailty, disability, and interprofessional collaboration.
7. Integrate an approach that respects the person's choices and values in the palliative and end of life stages.
8. Evaluate the impact of palliative dental hygiene oral care on the person.

SHORT ANSWER QUESTIONS

1. When are modifications made to standard of oral hygiene care in patients under palliative care?

_____

_____

_____

_____

2. Which classification of oral candidiasis includes elevated yellowish patches that cannot be wiped off?

_____

_____

_____

_____

3. Which classification of oral candidiasis includes elevated yellowish patches that can be wiped off?

_____

_____

_____

_____

4. Why would patients with xerostomia want to avoid products that contain lemon, glycerin, or alcohol?

_____

_____

_____

_____

5. What does the acronym REMAP stand for?

_____

_____

_____

_____

_____

FILL IN THE BLANK STATEMENTS

Select the best term from the chapter and complete the following statements.

1. _____ focuses on decreasing severity and symptoms of disease in patients with terminal diseases rather than delaying or reversing disease progression.

2. _____ focuses on patients' immediate comfort through management and prevention of oral complications caused by terminal disease process.

3. _____ is the time during which a patient copes with declining health from a terminal disease.

4. _____ occurs as white and red fissures in the commissures of the mouth.

5. _____ is another term for inability to swallow.

MULTIPLE CHOICE QUESTIONS

Complete each question by circling the best answer.

1. Hospice is a facility that patients with terminal diseases reside. Hospice provides compassion, support, and care for those in the last phases of terminal illness.
   a. Both statements are true.
   b. Both statements are false.
   c. The first statement is true, the second statement is false.
   d. The first statement is false, the second statement is true.

2. Oral health status free from pain and malodor contributes to all of the following EXCEPT:
   a. Prevent further decline in overall health
   b. Social interaction and communication
   c. Maintain nutritional intake
   d. Self-esteem

3. All of the following are oral complications found inpatients in palliative care EXCEPT:
   a. Candidiasis
   b. Macroglossia
   c. Mucositis
   d. Xerostomia

4. All of the following are classifications of oral candidiasis EXCEPT:
   a. Hyperplastic
   b. Pseudomembranous
   c. Erythematous
   d. Xerostomia

5. All of the following are characteristics of mucositis EXCEPT:
   a. Edematous tissue
   b. Burning sensation
   c. Trismus
   d. Yellow membrane covered ulcerations

6. The dental hygiene diagnosis will not change in a patient in palliative care because oral care stays the same once a patient reaches the need for palliative care.
   a. Both statements are true.
   b. Both statements are false.
   c. The first statement is true, the second statement is false.
   d. The first statement is false, the second statement is true.

7. The most important aspects of planning palliative oral care is pain management and:
   a. Hydration
   b. Keeping the dentition plaque free
   c. Completing any restoration needed as soon as possible
   d. Scaling and root debriding

8. Your patient with end-stage cancer presents with pain and as abscess associated with tooth number 9. She would prefer to have the tooth treated endodontically rather than extracting the tooth, to prevent any change in her appearance. What Human Needs Deficit does this address?
   a. Protection from Health Risks
   b. Freedom from Pain
   c. Wholesome Facial Image
   d. Skin and Mucous Membrane Integrity of the Head and Neck

9. Concerning question 8, what Human Needs deficit would be addressed if the patient preferred to have the tooth removed and was not concerned about appearance?
   a. Protection from Health Risks
   b. Freedom from Pain
   c. Wholesome Facial Image
   d. Skin and Mucous Membrane Integrity of the Head and Neck

10. All of the following are common antifungal agents used to treat candidiasis EXCEPT:
    a. Miconazole 2%
    b. Clotrimazole 1%
    c. Nystatin
    d. Amoxicillin 500 mg

CASE STUDY

Your patient, a 90-year-old resident of a long-term care facility, has pancreatic cancer and is not expected to live beyond 3 months. She reports that her full maxillary denture does not fit well and has a bad taste. She also reports pain on her palate. She also wears a partial mandibular denture and has maintained the teeth she has left diligently over the past several years. Oral exam reveals angular cheilitis and pseudomembranous candidiasis on the palate. Develop a dental hygiene diagnosis and care plan that includes goals and interventions. What education concepts would you use? What is the priority for this patient?

_____

_____

_____

_____

_____

_____

_____

_____

_____

_____

_____

_____

_____

53 Autoimmune Diseases

COMPETENCIES

1. Explain immune dysfunction.
2. Describe the pathophysiology of autoimmune diseases.
3. Describe pharmacologic considerations for autoimmune diseases.
4. Implement the dental hygiene process of care for patients presenting with autoimmune diseases, including:
   - Recognize the systemic and oral manifestations of common autoimmune diseases.
   - Develop a dental hygiene care plan appropriate for persons with autoimmune disease.
   - Deliver dental hygiene services safely and effectively for patients with autoimmune disease.

SHORT ANSWER QUESTIONS

1. Name the two factors that are necessary for autoimmune progress.

   _____

   _____

   _____

2. Name the two paths of tissue destruction due to autoimmune diseases.

   _____

   _____

   _____

3. Briefly describe the characteristics of multiple sclerosis.

   _____

   _____

   _____

   _____

4. List risk assessment tools for those with autoimmune disorders.

   _____

   _____

   _____

   _____

5. What are the oral manifestations of pemphigoid and what is the treatment?

   _____

   _____

   _____

   _____

354

Chapter **53** Autoimmune Diseases

FILL IN THE BLANK STATEMENTS

Select the best term from the chapter and complete the following statements.

1. _____ demonstrates patient's comfort in managing daily activities of living related to oral health.

2. Autoimmune disease treatment begins with _____ medications and progresses to _____ medications.

3. A disease in which injury is caused mainly by deposition of immune complexes and binding of antibodies to various cells and tissues, and affects major organ systems characterized by periods of remissions and exacerbations, is _____

4. _____ levels are highest in the morning, which helps ensure patient safety by minimizing risks for adrenal crisis.

5. Patients with _____ may experience pathologic jaw fractures late in the disease process.

MULTIPLE CHOICE QUESTIONS

Complete each question by circling the best answer.

1. The first agent of choice in treating rheumatoid arthritis is:
   a. Salicylates
   b. Acetaminophen
   c. Opiates
   d. Anticholinergics

2. Which drug prevents joint and tissue damage in those with rheumatoid arthritis?
   a. Salicylates
   b. DMARD
   c. NSAIDS
   d. Cyclosporine

3. All of the following medications contribute adverse bleeding events EXCEPT:
   a. COX-2
   b. NSAIDS
   c. Salicylates
   d. Acetaminophen

4. All of the following oral side effects may occur with patients receiving long-term corticosteroid therapy EXCEPT:
   a. Candidiasis
   b. Xerostomia
   c. Gingival hyperplasia
   d. Slow wound healing

5. Which autoimmune disease manifests with decrease in acetylcholine receptors in muscle fibers, resulting in progressive fatigability and abnormality of skeletal muscles?
   a. Psoriasis
   b. Fibromyalgia
   c. Hyperthyroidism
   d. Myasthenia gravis

6. Which autoimmune disease manifests connective tissue secondary to vascular injury and progressive interstitial and perivascular fibrosis of the skin and multiple organs?
   a. Scleroderma
   b. Hypothyroidism
   c. Psoriasis
   d. Lupus

7. Your patient reports with oral manifestations of pernicious anemia that include painful, red, burning tongue with atrophy of papillae. What is the BEST Human Needs Conceptual model deficit?
   a. Protection from Health Risks
   b. Freedom from Fear and Stress
   c. Freedom from Pain
   d. Wholesome Facial Image

8. All of the following are autoimmune diseases EXCEPT:
   a. Glaucoma
   b. Fibromyalgia
   c. Psoriasis
   d. Rheumatoid arthritis

9. Which of the following treatment creates the greatest stressor that leads to excessive cortisol secretion?
   a. Local anesthesia delivery
   b. Surgery
   c. Periodontal therapy
   d. ER visit

10. An enlarged tongue is a manifestation of what autoimmune disease?
   a. Pernicious anemia
   b. Scleroderma
   c. Sjögren's Syndrome
   d. Hypothyroidism

11. Which medication causes delayed would healing, osteoporosis, weight gain, and peptic ulcers with chronic use?
    a. Acetaminophen
    b. Methotrexate
    c. Corticosteroids
    d. NSAIDS

12. Which medication may cause blue-black lesions of the oral mucosa?
    a. Salicylates
    b. DMARDS
    c. COX-2 inhibitors
    d. Cyclosporine

13. Which of the following are oral manifestations found with psoriasis?
    a. Gingival bleeding
    b. Rapid onset of periodontal disease
    c. Anterior open bite
    d. Oral manifestations are rare

CASE STUDY

Your patient, a 38-year-old female, presents for her routine dental hygiene care appointment and was last seen 6 months ago. You notice today that her eyelids are drooping slightly. She reports that she cannot swallow or chew well. As she is speaking, her mouth appears to have difficulty forming words. What condition do you suspect you patient has developed? What medical interventions does she need? What dental hygiene interventions will you plan?

_____

_____

_____

_____

_____

_____

_____

_____

_____

_____

_____

_____

_____

_____

_____

_____

_____

COMPETENCIES

1. Explain the concept of solid organ transplantation, discuss the indications for organ transplantation, and describe the role that the United Network for Organ Sharing (UNOS) plays in organ transplantation.
2. Determine specialized dental management considerations of patients' oral health needs before solid organ transplantation and after transplantation.
3. Discuss the world-recognized Kidney Disease Outcomes Quality Initiative (K/DOQI), as well as compare and contrast chronic kidney disease and end-stage renal disease.
4. Discuss dialysis treatment modalities.
5. Describe various secondary medical conditions that could develop with kidney disease and dialysis and relate these conditions to overall oral care.
6. Discuss the need for interprofessional communication among members of the transplant patient's medical healthcare team.

SHORT ANSWER QUESTIONS

1. What systemic factors increase the risk of developing chronic kidney disease?

_____

_____

_____

_____

2. Briefly describe the five stages of chronic renal failure.

_____

_____

_____

_____

_____

3. What are the complications of patients with all stages of kidney disease?

_____

_____

_____

_____

_____

_____

4. Why would a patient with end-stage renal disease have dental erosion on anterior teeth?

_____

_____

_____

_____

5. What are the two types of uremic stomatitis?

_____

_____

_____

_____

_____

_____

_____

_____

_____

FILL IN THE BLANK STATEMENTS

Select the best term from the chapter and complete the following statements.

1. _____ is the surgical placement of a viable functioning organ in a patient with end-stage organ disease.

2. Organ donation received from a living relative donor is _____

3. Organ donation received from an unrelated person is _____

4. Organ donation received from a twin donor is _____

5. _____ is a nonprofit organization that is the only organ network.

6. _____ is a noxious effect of some substances, toxic chemicals and medications, on renal function.

7. _____ is altered or impaired taste perception that often includes metallic taste.

8. _____ is itchy skin in patients with end-stage renal disease.

MULTIPLE CHOICE QUESTIONS

Complete each question by circling the best answer.

1. During extraoral exam of your patient with end-stage renal disease, you observe white patches of skin on the face and arms. This is most likely:
   a. Uremic eczema
   b. Uremic frost
   c. Pityriasis alba
   d. Milia

2. Patients with liver transplants have a increased incidence of all of the following EXCEPT:
   a. Basal cell carcinoma
   b. Oropharyngeal cancer
   c. Lung cancer
   d. Squamous cell carcinoma

3. All of the following are gastrointestinal clinical manifestations of chronic renal disease EXCEPT:
   a. Hepatitis
   b. Anorexia
   c. Reflux
   d. Peptic ulcer

4. Transplant recipients commonly receive all of the following long-term immunosuppressive medications EXCEPT:
   a. Tacrolimus
   b. Cyclosporine
   c. Prednisone
   d. Mycophenolate mofetil

5. Organ transplant recipients should always receive antibiotic premedication prior to invasive dental procedures. Organ transplant recipients should always be medically evaluated to determine if or when they may receive routine dental care.
   a. Both statements are true.
   b. Both statements are false.
   c. The first statement is true, the second statement is false.
   d. The first statement is false, the second statement is true.

6. The most current test to accurately measure renal function is:
   a. CT scan
   b. Alanine transaminase test
   c. Glomerular filtration rate
   d. Abdominal ultrasound

7. Primary treatment goal of a patient with chronic renal failure is to reduce the risk of:
   a. CVD
   b. Diabetes
   c. Malnutrition
   d. Anemia

8. A disease that causes inflammation of the glomeruli or the kidney's filtering units is called:
   a. Glomerulonephritis
   b. Hemodialysis
   c. Nephritis
   d. Pyelonephritis

9. All of the following are cardiovascular clinical manifestations of chronic renal disease EXCEPT:
   a. Pericarditis
   b. Atherosclerosis
   c. Hypertension
   d. Mycobacterial infection

10. All of the following are oral clinical manifestations of chronic renal disease EXCEPT:
    a. Enamel hyperplasia
    b. Fungal infection
    c. Saliva has ammonia odor
    d. Pale mucosa

11. Chronic kidney disease is a gradual loss of function that reduces the ability of kidneys to:
    a. Absorb water
    b. Metabolize calcium
    c. Filter blood
    d. Filter urine

CASE STUDY: MR. WASHINGTON

A 35-year-old African American male presented to your office for dental clearance as a requirement for placement on kidney transplant list. The patient has been on hemodialysis since January 2012. Patient has end-stage renal failure. The patient reports moderate anxiety when receiving dental treatment. No reported allergies.

Age	35	SCENARIO
Gender	male	**EOE IOE** Oral mucosa pale. Some areas of slight maxillary lingual erosion.
Height	5'11"	**Periodontal** Generalized moderate to severe periodontal disease with pocket depths of 5-6 mm pocketing and 2-3 mm recession. Generalized heavy supra- and subcalculus with heavy biofilm #23-26 class III mobility with poor prognosis
Weight	210 lb	**Radiographic** 2-3 mm of horizontal bone loss evident.
B/P	155/85 mm Hg	**Dental** Decay in occlusal surfaces of all molars, #15 hopeless, will need extraction #23-26 extract and replace with partial denture
Chief Complaint	Dental clearance as a requirement for placement on kidney transplant list Intermittent pain max posterior bilateral Gums are sore and bleed	
Medical History Current Medications	Patient reports dialysis delivered through a fistula on the left lower forearm since 2012, delivered on M-W-F schedule. A medical consult was requested with his primary care physician to determine if the patient needed premedication. His physician suggested a premedication of 2 g Amoxicillin one hour prior to treatment. Aciphex 20 mg as needed for acid reflux Catapres .2 mg for hypertension; during hemodialysis Epogen 2200 units IV Fosrenol 1000 mg Heparin 6000 units IV Lisinopril 10 mg and Minoxidil 10 mg for hypertension Mobic 7.5 mg to prevent bone disease Nephro-Vite one tablet daily Normodyne 200 mg 2×/day Sensipar 60 mg for hyperparathyroidism in dialysis patients	Approximately 5 years since his last dental visit, the patient presents only for emergency care. Patient reports pain in posterior teeth, bleeding and sore gums when brushing, uses medium toothbrush once a day and does not use floss.
Social History	Non-drinker Non-smoker Former heroin addict	

Using the data from this patient, develop a Human Needs Conceptual model for treatment.

Dental Hygiene Diagnosis (unmet human need)	Etiology (due to…)	Signs and Symptoms (evidenced by…)	Patient Goals (expected outcomes)
Protection from Health Risks			
Freedom from Fear and Stress			
Freedom from Pain			
Wholesome Facial Image			
Skin and Mucous Membrane Integrity of the Head and Neck			
Biologically Sound and Functional Dentition			
Conceptualization and Problem Solving			
Responsibility for Oral Health			

Develop a treatment plan for this patient. Include a schedule, type of anesthesia to be used and why, oral hygiene education, and recommendations. What members of Mr. Washington's interprofessional team would you contact and why? What further information would you need to begin treatment?

_____

_____

_____

_____

_____

_____

_____

_____

_____

_____

_____

_____

_____

_____

55 Respiratory Diseases

COMPETENCIES

1. Discuss the etiology, risk factors, signs and symptoms, and related medications associated with asthma and chronic obstructive pulmonary disease (COPD) as they relate to the process of dental hygiene care. Develop a dental hygiene care plan applicable for a person with either asthma or COPD, addressing adaptations needed for the specific respiratory disease.
2. Discuss the etiology, risk factors, signs and symptoms, and related medications of tuberculosis as they relate to the process of dental hygiene care. Develop a dental hygiene care plan applicable for a person with tuberculosis, addressing adaptations needed for the disease.
3. Discuss the etiology and types of pneumonia as they relate to the process of dental hygiene care. Develop a dental hygiene care plan applicable for a person with pneumonia, and relate the role of a dental hygienist to caring for the infirmed or intubated patient, as well as educate other healthcare providers involved in oral care to prevent pneumonia.
4. Apply knowledge of sleep-related breathing disorders to assessment, care planning, and treatment implementation by dental hygienists and other oral healthcare providers.

SHORT ANSWER QUESTIONS

1. List medications that are contraindicated in patients with asthma.

_____

_____

_____

_____

2. Describe signs and symptoms of an acute asthma attack.

_____

_____

_____

_____

_____

_____

3. Describe causes of global tuberculosis incidence.

_____

_____

_____

_____

_____

_____

_____

4. What are the symptoms of acute tuberculosis?

_____

_____

_____

_____

5. What are the two subcategories of pneumonia?

_____

_____

6. What are the risk factors of CAP?

_____

_____

_____

7. What are the risk factors of VAP?

_____

_____

_____

_____

_____

_____

8. What are the characteristics of sleep apnea?

_____

_____

_____

_____

_____

_____

_____

9. What are the oral manifestations of sleep apnea?

_____

_____

_____

_____

_____

_____

FILL IN THE BLANK STATEMENTS

Select the best term from the chapter and complete the following statements.

1. Difficulty breathing is also known as _____.

2. _____ is a hyperinflation of lungs and irreversible destruction of lung tissue.

3. _____ is a condition characterized by spasms in the bronchi of the lungs, causing difficulty in breathing as a response to various stimuli, allergy, or other forms of hypersensitivity.

4. _____ is a lung disease, marked by limitations of lung airflow caused by noxious substances, that interferes with normal breathing and is not fully reversible.

5. _____ is a mucus-producing cough and expectoration that is prevalent 3 out of 12 months for 2 consecutive years with no underlying disease.

6. _____ is an airborne communicable disease that affects lungs as well as other organs and tissues.

7. _____ is a lung inflammation caused by bacterial or viral infection, in which the air sacs fill with exudate and may solidify.

8. Difficulty swallowing is also known as _____.

9. _____ occurs when there is a partial or complete collapse of airway and breathing during sleep.

MULTIPLE CHOICE QUESTIONS

Complete each question by circling the best answer.

1. During an asthma attack, blood pressure, pulse, respiration, and temperature increase. Asthma is an acute inflammatory response disease.
   a. Both statements are true.
   b. Both statements are false.
   c. The first statement is true, the second statement is false.
   d. The first statement is false, the second statement is true.

2. The major risk factor for COPD is:
   a. Cigarette smoking
   b. Asbestos exposure
   c. Untreated chronic bronchitis
   d. Uncontrolled asthma

3. Which of the following respiratory diseases may have a genetic predisposition?
   a. Chronic bronchitis
   b. Asthma
   c. COPD
   d. Emphysema

4. Nitrous oxide is contraindicated for patients with which respiratory disease?
   a. Asthma
   b. COPD
   c. Chronic bronchitis
   d. Emphysema

5. Air polishing is contraindicated for patients with which respiratory disease?
   a. Asthma
   b. Chronic bronchitis
   c. Emphysema
   d. COPD

6. Patients with latent TB infections are contagious. Latent TB infection includes low-grade fever, cough, and malaise.
   a. Both statements are true.
   b. Both statements are false.
   c. The first statement is true, the second statement is false.
   d. The first statement is false, the second statement is true.

7. What is the most important aspect of treating a patient with a history of TB?
   a. How long ago was the infection
   b. Correct medication was taken
   c. Risk of transmission
   d. Medication regiment was completed

8. Over half of all CAP cases are bacterial infections. The most common organism that causes pneumonia is *Staphylococcus pneumonia.*
   a. Both statements are true.
   b. Both statements are false.
   c. The first statement is true, the second statement is false.
   d. The first statement is false, the second statement is true.

9. All of the following are subcategories of nosocomial pneumonia EXCEPT:
   a. Hospital acquired
   b. Ventilator associated
   c. Healthcare associated
   d. Aspiration associated

10. All of the following medications are contraindicated for patients with asthma EXCEPT:
    a. Aspirin
    b. Narcotics
    c. Penicillins
    d. NSAIDS

CASE STUDY: MRS. GREENE

Develop a treatment plan for this patient. Describe what type of comprehensive treatment you would implement. What treatment is contraindicated in this patient? What considerations would you make?

Address chair position, salivary flow, candidiasis, consult with interprofessional team member.

Age	60	SCENARIO
Gender	female	**EOE/IOE:** candidiasis present on tongue and palate
Height	5'6"	
Weight	120 lb	
B/P	110/72 mm Hg	**Periodontal Findings:** Probe readings 3-4 mm generalized with 1-mm recession generalized
Chief Complaint	Dry mouth Roof of mouth and tongue is sore	
Medical History	COPD	Generalized moderate biofilm with slight calculus on mandibular anterior teeth Moderate BOP generalized
Current Medications	Beclovent daily Flonase daily Prednisone 10 mg daily Albuterol as needed Singulair 20 mg daily	**Radiographic Findings:** WNL **Dental Findings:** WNL
Social History	Social drinker Smokes ½ pack of cigarettes daily Occasionally smokes marijuana	

56 Substance Use Disorders

COMPETENCIES

1. Describe concepts of substance use disorders and mental illness.
2. Discuss concepts of illicit and over-the-counter drug use, including drug schedules, club drugs, marijuana, and the opioid crisis in the United States.
3. Explain which medical treatments are used for various substance abuses.
4. Analyze the dental hygiene process of care related to patients with substance use disorders and those in recovery.
5. Discuss why dental professionals may be at risk for substance use disorders.

SHORT ANSWER QUESTIONS

1. What are the social consequences of substance misuse?
   a. Alcohol- or drug-impaired drivers cause a significant number of deadly automobile accidents
   b. Child abuse and neglect
   c. Intimate partner violence
   d. Sexual violence
   e. Suicide attempts and fatalities, overdose deaths
   f. Various forms of cancer
   g. Heart and liver diseases
   h. Human immunodeficiency virus (HIV) / acquired immunodeficiency disease syndrome (AIDS)
   i. Fetal alcohol spectrum disorders (FASDs)
   j. Neonatal abstinence syndrome (NAS)

2. Give examples of club drugs.
    a. Methylenedioxymethamphetamine (MDMA)
    b. Gamma-hydroxybutyrate (GHB)
    c. Ketamine
    d. Rohypnol
    e. Methamphetamine
    f. Lysergic Acid Diethylamide (LSD)

_____

_____

_____

_____

_____

_____

_____

_____

_____

_____

3. What are the overdose symptoms of depressants?
    a. Dilated pupils
    b. Shallow breathing
    c. Weak or rapid pulse
    d. Clammy skin
    e. Coma

_____

_____

_____

_____

_____

_____

_____

_____

_____

_____

4. What are the overdose symptoms of narcotics?
   a. Clammy skin
   b. Convulsions
   c. Coma
   d. Slow, shallow breathing

   _____

   _____

   _____

   _____

   _____

   _____

   _____

   _____

5. What are typical oral findings of a person who uses amphetamines?
   a. Xerostomia
   b. Increased caries
   c. Bruxism
   d. Trismus

   _____

   _____

   _____

   _____

   _____

   _____

   _____

6. What are typical oral findings of a person who uses marijuana?
   a. Leukoplakia
   b. Increased incidence of lingual carcinoma
   c. Gingival enlargement

   _____

   _____

   _____

   _____

   _____

7. What are the symptoms of alcohol poisoning?
   a. Slow or irregular breathing (<8 breaths per minute)
   b. Cold, pale, or blue-toned skin
   c. Rapid pulse
   d. Vomiting while awake or asleep
   e. Unresponsive to attempts to awaken
   f. Semiconsciousness or unconsciousness

_____

_____

_____

_____

_____

_____

_____

_____

_____

8. List how various drugs may enter the body.
   a. Direct contact with skin or mucous membranes
   b. Swallowing
   c. Snorted through the nose
   d. Placed sublingually
   e. Placed against oral mucosa
   f. Injected directly into the bloodstream (intravenously)
   g. Injected into a muscle (muscling)
   h. Injected under the skin (skin popping)

_____

_____

_____

_____

_____

_____

_____

_____

_____

_____

371

FILL IN THE BLANK STATEMENTS

Select the best term from the chapter and complete the following statements.

1. _____ is the prolonged, repeated misuse of any substance – a chronic and compulsive need to use drugs despite their causing the user physical harm.

2. _____ are substance classifications in relation to their acceptable medical use and the misuse or dependency potential.

3. _____ are substances that are used nonmedical purposes and are illegal to manufacture, use, or sell.

4. _____ are available for purchase without a prescription, have psychoactive or mind-altering properties that can lead to serious medical and mental health conditions

5. _____ is a biologic alteration in the user's brain from consistent drug use.

6. _____ in the belief that the drug is needed to maintain a state of well-being.

7. _____ is a pattern of self-administered drug use that may lead to addiction.

8. _____ is the increasingly larger dose required to produce the same physiological or psychological effect obtained earlier with smaller doses.

9. A person who has developed physiological dependence on a drug will go through drug _____ when drug use stops.

10. _____ are group of psychoactive drugs that act on the central nervous system and cause changes in mood, awareness, and behavior and are often misused by young adults.

MULTIPLE CHOICE QUESTIONS

Complete each question by circling the best answer.

1. All of the following are the three main types of alcohol EXCEPT:
   a. Methanol
   b. Ethanol
   c. Isopropyl
   d. Ethylene glycol

2. Ecstasy and peyote are Schedule I drugs. Tylenol with codeine, tramadol and valium are Schedule III drugs
   a. Both statements are true.
   b. Both statements are false.
   c. The first statement is true and the second statement is false.
   d. The first statement is false and the second statement is true.

3. All of the following are systemic effects of anabolic steroid use EXCEPT:
   a. Low blood pressure
   b. Tremors
   c. Depression
   d. Acne

4. Long-term use of alcohol may lead to hepatitis, malnutrition and dementia. Systemic effects of alcohol use may lead to cognitive impairment, cirrhosis of the lover and damage to kidneys.
   a. Both statements are true.
   b. Both statements are false.
   c. The first statement is true and the second statement is false.
   d. The first statement is false and the second statement is true.

5. Fermenting simple carbohydrates produces ethanol. Methanol is the most common alcohol found in alcoholic beverages.
   a. Both statements are true.
   b. Both statements are false.
   c. The first statement is true and the second statement is false.
   d. The first statement is false and the second statement is true.

6. What percent concentration of blood alcohol is illegal in most US jurisdictions?
   a. 0.01%
   b. 0.1%
   c. 1.0%
   d. 10%

7. Psychologically dependent addicts misuse substances to cope with life. With therapy, physically dependent addicts may be able to return to social use.
   a. Both statements are true.
   b. Both statements are false.
   c. The first statement is true and the second statement is false.
   d. The first statement is false and the second statement is true.

8. All of the following are short-term effects of marijuana EXCEPT:
   a. Feeling of euphoria
   b. Poor concentration
   c. Difficulty with problem solving
   d. Mild depression

9. When treating alcoholism, what is the mechanism of action of Antabuse?
   a. Decreases the craving for alcohol
   b. Blocks the metabolism of alcohol
   c. Eliminates the craving for alcohol
   d. Blocks serotonin receptors

10. All of the following are examples of illicit drugs EXCEPT:
   a. Codeine
   b. Cocaine
   c. Heroin
   d. Hallucinogens

11. Which of the following schedules of drug has the lowest potential for misuse or dependency?
   a. I
   b. II
   c. IV
   d. V

12. A physically dependent addict displays all of the following behaviors EXCEPT:
   a. Withdrawal signs
   b. Not used as a coping device
   c. Does not result in personal problems
   d. Adapts to the body's chemistry

Angus has been a long-time patient in your office. He is a successful sales manager for a luxury car lot. Angus has made no secret that he excessively drinks alcohol and considers himself a functioning alcoholic. He states he has been a heavy drinker for many years, why stop now? He states that he was recently hospitalized for a skin infection. He admits to not eating healthy and often skips meals altogether. His oral health has severely declined over the last 2 years and you are concerned that he is not understanding the implications of alcohol use on his oral health and overall health.

Age	62	SCENARIO
Gender	male	**EOE/IOE:**
Height	6'	Enamel erosion evident on all maxillary lingual tooth surfaces
Weight	200 lb	Heavy biofilm generalized
B/P	130/80 mm Hg	Moderate calculus generalized
Chief Complaint	"my mouth feels dry a lot" "I broke a tooth but don't remember how it happened. It's a little sensitive"	Glossitis Coated tongue Moderate attrition on anterior teeth
Medical History	Asthma	**Periodontal Findings:** 5-6 mm pockets posterior teeth, 3-4 mm pockets anterior teeth
Current Medications	Proventil inhaler prn	2 mm recession generalized Generalized moderate BOP
Social History	Heavy alcohol drinker – reports drinking 4-6 whiskey drinks a day 4 oz each Smokes an occasional cigar about 1 per week	**Radiographic Findings:** #3 MOD caries #4 DO caries #15 MO caries #30 O caries **Dental Findings:** #10 incisal edge chipped with slight sensitivity #23-26 class I mobility

1. What is your dental hygiene diagnosis for Angus?
2. Develop a dental hygiene care plan including goals and interventions
3. What patient education issues should be addressed?
4. What factors could be contributing to this patient's periodontal health?

Using the data from this patient, develop a Human Needs Conceptual model for treatment.

Dental Hygiene Diagnosis (unmet human need)	Etiology (due to…)	Signs and Symptoms (evidenced by…)	Patient Goals (expected outcomes)
Protection from Health Risks			
Freedom from Fear and Stress			
Freedom from Pain			
Wholesome Facial Image			
Skin and Mucous Membrane Integrity of the Head and Neck			
Biologically Sound and Functional Dentition			
Conceptualization and Problem Solving			
Responsibility for Oral Health			

57 Eating Disorders

COMPETENCIES

1. Describe the diagnosis and epidemiology of both anorexia nervosa and bulimia nervosa.
2. Discuss oral and overall health effects of anorexia nervosa and bulimia nervosa.
3. Develop a dental hygiene care plan for a patient with an eating disorder that includes (a) engaging the patient in a dialogue of disclosure of an eating disorder, (b) assessing oral health needs, (c) planning for reduction of harm and promotion of oral health, (d) implementing dental-hygiene interventions, and (e) evaluating outcomes of care.
4. Discuss the need for interprofessional collaboration for patient-centered care of a patient with an eating disorder.
5. List resources available to help patients with eating disorders.

SHORT ANSWER QUESTIONS

1. List primary medical symptoms of anorexia nervosa.

_____

_____

_____

_____

_____

_____

_____

2. List oral findings of patients with eating disorders.

_____

_____

_____

_____

_____

_____

_____

3. List primary medical symptoms of bulimia.

_____

_____

_____

_____

_____

_____

_____

4. What are the two most common physical findings of a patient with advanced anorexia nervosa?

_____

_____

_____

_____

5. When discussing suspected eating disorder with a patient who has anorexia nervosa or bulimia, common responses are:

_____

_____

_____

_____

_____

FILL IN THE BLANK STATEMENTS

Select the best term from the chapter and complete the following statements.

1. Two types of bulimia are _____ and _____.

2. Enamel erosion is also known as _____.

3. Very thin, soft, unpigmented, downy hair is also known as _____.

4. _____ is s a hormone that is produced and released by the stomach with small amounts also released by the small intestine, pancreas, and brain and is considered the 'hunger hormone' because it stimulates appetite, increases food intake, and promotes fat storage.

5. _____ is an eating disorder characterized by weight loss with difficulties maintaining an appropriate body weight for height, age, and stature and a distorted body image.

MULTIPLE CHOICE QUESTIONS

Complete each question by circling the best answer.

1. The criteria for diagnosing anorexia includes all of the following findings EXCEPT:
   a. Extreme restrictive food intake
   b. Intense fear of gaining weight
   c. Lack of serious concern for current weight
   d. Repeated self-induced vomiting of at least one month

2. The teeth and surfaces that are affected by bulimia nervosa first are:
   a. Maxillary anterior lingual
   b. Maxillary posterior lingual
   c. Mandibular anterior lingual
   d. Mandibular posterior lingual

3. The first phase of treatment planning in a patient with a suspected eating disorder is:
   a. Treat and stabilize periodontal condition
   b. Restore areas of decay as a result of erosion
   c. Refer to medical and psychological providers
   d. Educate patient on various treatments for sensitivity

4. All of the following are recommendations to patients who induce vomiting EXCEPT:
   a. Daily fluoride
   b. Brushing directly after vomiting
   c. Neutralize oral acidity after vomiting
   d. Using a mouth guard during vomiting

5. When assessing a patient with suspected or previously diagnosed eating disorder, the most common assessment technique used is:
   a. Collaborative consultation
   b. Interview
   c. Intraoral exam
   d. Observation

6. A patient that presents to your office with a diagnosis with anorexia nervosa is considered medically compromised. This patient is not psychiatrically compromised, however.
   a. Both statements are true.
   b. Both statements are false.
   c. The first statement is true, the second statement is false.
   d. The first statement is false, the second statement is true.

7. Many patients who have an eating disorder often seek dental care due to sensitivity from purging. Eating disorders affect multiple systemic functions.
   a. Both statements are true.
   b. Both statements are false.
   c. The first statement is true, the second statement is false.
   d. The first statement is false, the second statement is true.

8. Collaboration between dental professionals and specific eating disorder healthcare providers increases success of interventions. Strong evidence supports how eating disorders affect oral health.
   a. Both statements are true.
   b. Both statements are false.
   c. The first statement is true, the second statement is false.
   d. The first statement is false, the second statement is true.

9. All of the following are oral manifestations of eating disorders EXCEPT:
   a. Parotid gland enlargement
   b. Hypersalivation
   c. Perimylolysis
   d. Dental hypersensitivity

10. A 20-year-old female patient presents with signs and symptoms that may indicate an eating disorder. What Human Needs Conceptual model deficits would this address?
    a. Wholesome Facial Image
    b. Skin and Mucous Membrane Integrity of the Head and Neck
    c. Protection from Health Risks
    d. Conceptualization and Problem Solving

CASE STUDY: MS. HEATH

Age	21	SCENARIO
Gender	female	**EOE/IOE:**
Height	5'4"	Enlarged parotid glands
Weight	95 lb	Erosion on many teeth
B/P	100/50 mm Hg	Oral tissues dehydrated
		Xerostomia
Chief Complaint	Sensitivity, tooth discoloration, pain	
Medical History	Anorexia nervosa	**Periodontal Findings:**
		Generalized bleeding, inflammation, bulbous tissues
Current Medications	Prozac	Slight horizontal bone loss around molars
Social History	Non-drinker	**Radiographic Findings:**
	Non-smoker	Rampant caries
		Dental Findings:
		Several areas of decay
		Other Observations:
		Very dry skin
		Lack of communication concerning health

Using the data from this patient, develop a Human Needs Conceptual model for treatment.

Dental Hygiene Diagnosis (unmet human need)	Etiology (due to…)	Signs and Symptoms (evidenced by…)	Patient Goals (expected outcomes)
Protection from Health Risks			
Freedom from Fear and Stress			
Freedom from Pain			
Wholesome Facial Image			
Skin and Mucous Membrane Integrity of the Head and Neck			
Biologically Sound and Functional Dentition			
Conceptualization and Problem Solving			
Responsibility for Oral Health			

Develop a care plan for Ms. Heath. Include any interprofessional interventions.

58 Child Abuse and Neglect and Family Violence

1. Apply knowledge of indicators of abuse and neglect in clinical patient care and utilize social support and public health resources to report and assist victims of family violence and human trafficking.
2. Incorporate assessment of abuse and neglect among child, adult, elderly, vulnerable adults, and victims of human trafficking as a routine part of the dental hygiene visit.
3. Collaborate with interprofessional healthcare providers in the education, early detection, and early intervention for victims of child maltreatment, intimate partner violence, elder and vulnerable adult abuse and neglect, and human trafficking.
4. Assume primary prevention and advocacy roles in educating patients, communities, and professional colleagues in health, law, and social support services regarding dental findings associated with abuse and neglect.
5. Explain the links between child maltreatment and intimate partner violence and bullying and the power and control demonstrated by perpetrators of family violence and neglect and human trafficking.

SHORT ANSWER QUESTIONS

1. What is PANDA? Briefly explain.

_____

_____

_____

_____

2. List examples of oral health findings of a person who is or has been neglected.

_____

_____

_____

_____

_____

_____

_____

_____

_____

3. List examples of findings of a person who is or has been sexually abused.

_____

_____

_____

_____

_____

_____

_____

_____

4. List examples of findings of a person who is or has been emotionally abused.

_____

_____

_____

_____

_____

_____

5. List examples of oral health findings of a person who is or has been physically abused.

_____

_____

_____

_____

_____

_____

_____

_____

_____

_____

_____

_____

_____

FILL IN THE BLANK STATEMENTS

Select the best term from the chapter and complete the following statements.

1. _____ is to treat a person with cruelty or violence regularly or repeatedly, also known as_____.

2. _____ is a caretaker's failure to provide care with proper food, clothing, shelter, supervision, medical care, or emotional stability.

3. _____ are also known as condyloma acuminatum.

4. _____ is the use of force or coercion to abuse or intimidate others.

5. _____ is abusive behavior used by a current or former partner to gain or maintain power and control over another intimate partner.

6. _____ is a crime where humans are treated as merchandise and bought and sold for profit.

MULTIPLE CHOICE QUESTIONS

Complete each question by circling the best answer.

1. The age group with the highest incidence of child maltreatment is:
   a. Birth to 12 months
   b. 13 months-24 months
   c. 2-4 years
   d. 5-7 years

2. The most prevalent reported type of child maltreatment is:
   a. Physical
   b. Emotional
   c. Sexual
   d. Neglect

3. The most common area of the body that incurs over half of the reported cases of child maltreatment is:
   a. Genital
   b. Head
   c. Arms
   d. Buttocks

4. Victims of child sexual abuse most often know their abuser. Victims of child sexual abuse often confide in a friend or family member.
   a. Both statements are true.
   b. Both statements are false.
   c. The first statement is true and the second statement is false.
   d. The first statement is false and the second statement is true.

5. An abusive caregiver will delay seeking medical or dental care following an injury. A neglectful parent will miss numerous appointments.
   a. Both statements are true.
   b. Both statements are false.
   c. The first statement is true and the second statement is false.
   d. The first statement is false and the second statement is true.

6. The offenders of most elder abuse and neglect cases are:
   a. Nursing home employees
   b. Home healthcare workers
   c. Family members
   d. Random strangers

7. The most common type of elder maltreatment is:
   a. Physical
   b. Emotional
   c. Financial
   d. Neglect

8. Deprivation of food, water, medical care, shelter, and education is an example of:
   a. Physical abuse
   b. Sexual abuse
   c. Neglect
   d. Emotional abuse

9. Intimidation with gestures, yelling, threats, and isolation is an example of:
   a. Physical abuse
   b. Sexual abuse
   c. Neglect
   d. Emotional abuse

10. Fatalities associated with child maltreatment are highest in what age group?
    a. Birth to 3 years
    b. 4 to 6 years
    c. 7-9 years
    d. 10-13 years

11. All of the following genetic conditions may mimic signs of physical abuse EXCEPT:
    a. Sturge-Weber syndrome
    b. Idiopathic thrombocytopenic purpura
    c. Ehlers-Danlos syndrome
    d. Dentinogenesis imperfecta

12. Dental hygienists are mandated to report suspicious cases of child maltreatment to the local Child Protective Services agency. Immunity laws protect dental hygienists from civil or criminal penalties resulting from filing a confidential report of suspected abuse and/or neglect.
    a. Both statements are true.
    b. Both statements are false.
    c. The first statement is true and the second statement is false.
    d. The first statement is false and the second statement is true.

CASE STUDY: MS. CUDWORTH

Age	13	SCENARIO
Gender	female	**EOE/IOE:**
Height	5'2"	Erythema and petechiae of the palate
Weight	100 lb	Lesion on left vestibule 4 mm circumference with cauliflower-like masses
B/P	105/70 mm Hg	
Chief Complaint	Pain in her throat	Heavy biofilm generalized
Medical History Current Medications	Seasonal allergies	Bruising apparent on left cheek under left eye
Social History	None	**Periodontal Findings:** Probe readings 1-3 mm generalized Severe gingivitis Spontaneous bleeding
		Radiographic Findings: Several areas of decay
		Dental Findings:
		Other Observations: Patient is withdrawn, shy, cooperative
		Grandmother recently obtained custody from drug-addicted parent

Develop a care plan for this patient. What is the dental hygienist's responsibility legally in this case?

_____

_____

_____

_____

_____

_____

_____

_____

_____

_____

_____

_____

_____

Using the data from this patient, develop a Human Needs Conceptual model for treatment.

Dental Hygiene Diagnosis (unmet human need)	Etiology (due to…)	Signs and Symptoms (evidenced by…)	Patient Goals (expected outcomes)
Protection from Health Risks			
Freedom from Fear and Stress			
Freedom from Pain			
Wholesome Facial Image			
Skin and Mucous Membrane Integrity of the Head and Neck			
Biologically Sound and Functional Dentition			
Conceptualization and Problem Solving			
Responsibility for Oral Health			

59 Disability and Healthcare

COMPETENCIES

By the end of this chapter, the reader will be able to:

1. Define "disability" and acquire knowledge about major developments, or circumstances, affecting patients with disabilities.
2. Distinguish different classifications for patients with disabilities.
3. Consider and recommend means to address healthcare barriers, assistive devices, and oral self-care devices for patients with disabilities. Provide oral self-care education to patients with disabilities and their caregivers.
4. Explain how to use protective stabilization and patient-positioning techniques throughout the delivery of professional care.
5. Care for patients in wheelchairs and recommend opportunities to advocate for patients with disabilities.

SHORT ANSWER QUESTIONS

1. Which stage of exposure to disability refers to conditions traceable to a disease or trauma?

_____

_____

_____

_____

2. Why do some healthcare providers avoid interacting with patients who have disabilities?

_____

_____

_____

_____

3. What should the dental hygienist assess before using assistive oral self-care devices?

_____

_____

_____

_____

4. List ideal characteristics for customized oral self-care devices.

_____

_____

_____

_____

5. What method should be used when transferring a patient in a wheelchair to prevent injury to the dental hygienist?

_____

_____

_____

_____

FILL IN THE BLANK STATEMENTS

Select the best term from the chapter and complete the following statements.

1. A person with a physical or mental impairment that substantially limits major life activities is considered to have a

_____.

2. _____ puts the person first, not the disability.

3. _____ is years of life lost due to disability.

4. Informed consent is necessary when utilizing _____ during treatment.

MULTIPLE CHOICE QUESTIONS

Complete each question by circling the best answer.

1. Using people-first language, select the appropriate reference to a person with a disability.
   a. Muscular dystrophy patient
   b. Patient with muscular dystrophy

2. All of the following are disability classifications EXCEPT:
   a. Participation restrictions
   b. Impairments
   c. Activity limitations
   d. Special needs

3. All of the following are stages of exposure to disability EXCEPT:
   a. Gender-associated
   b. Developmental
   c. Congenital
   d. Acquired

4. The primary reason people with disabilities do not receive needed healthcare services is:
   a. Cost
   b. Location of services
   c. Lack of transportation
   d. Limited services offered

5. Using a mechanical or physical device that immobilizes patient movement is:
   a. Assistive technology
   b. Protective stabilization
   c. Illegal in many states
   d. Used with sedated patients

6. Major life activities include all of the following EXCEPT:
   a. Breathing
   b. Running
   c. Sitting
   d. Standing

7. Using a parent, caregiver, or healthcare provider to physically immobilize a patient is:
   a. Illegal
   b. Active stabilization
   c. Passive stabilization
   d. Protective stabilization

8. Using a device to physically immobilize a patient is:
   a. Active stabilization
   b. Passive stabilization
   c. Protective stabilization
   d. Not necessary if the patient is conscious

9. To prevent pressure injuries on patients who use wheelchairs, the dental hygienist should:
   a. Keep the patient in the wheelchair during treatment
   b. Apply medication to affected areas, as needed
   c. Reposition the patient every 20 minutes
   d. Use passive stabilization

10. The Human Needs Conceptual Model deficit that addresses sa safe wheelchair transfer with a patient who has muscular dystrophy would be:
   a. Protection from Health Risks
   b. Freedom from Fear and Stress
   c. Freedom from Pain
   d. Wholesome Facial Image

CASE STUDY: MRS. P

Using the following information, how would you plan treatment for this patient? What accommodations would you make for her in the office? What adjustments to homecare would you make?

Age	70	SCENARIO
Gender	female	
Height	5'5"	
Weight	160 lb	
B/P	130/80 mm Hg	
Chief Complaint	Halitosis, unable to brush with conventional TB, unable to floss	
Medical History

Current Medications | Parkinson's disease
Type II diabetes
Early dementia

Glipizide
Namenda
Levodopa | 2 years since pt's last dental hygiene appointment.

Tremors in hands, balance is unstable, joints sore

Probe depths are 4-6 mm gen with mod-severe inflammation. Heavy biofilm and calc gen. |
| Social History | Widowed, lives in an assisted living facility | |

_____

_____

_____

_____

_____

_____

_____

_____

_____

_____

_____

_____

_____

_____

60 Intellectually and Developmentally Challenged

COMPETENCIES

1. List and describe the levels of intellectual disabilities (IDs) and relate general characteristics and individual needs and abilities of patients within each category of intellectual disabilities to modifications recommended for self-care education.
2. Plan alterations in dental hygiene care based on common medical conditions and intellectual disabilities associated with Down syndrome and other intellectual or developmental conditions.
3. Discuss general theories and characteristics of autism spectrum disorder (ASD).
4. Select and use effective instructional strategies to manage communication barriers with a patient who has ASD.
5. Value educational interventions for a patient with intellectual disabilities, Down syndrome, and ASD, and discuss the legal and ethical aspects of treating patients with developmental and/or physical challenges.

SHORT ANSWER QUESTIONS

1. List common oral manifestations of patients with intellectual disabilities.

_____

_____

_____

_____

_____

_____

2. List oral manifestations of patients with Down Syndrome.

_____

_____

_____

_____

_____

_____

3. What is the most common serious medical condition among patients with Down syndrome?

_____

4. What is the most common thyroid problem in patients over age 30 with Down syndrome?

_____

5. Give examples of clinical strategies for patients with autism.

_____

_____

_____

_____

_____

_____

6. List approaches to managing patients with autism.

_____

_____

_____

_____

_____

_____

FILL IN THE BLANK STATEMENTS

Select the best term from the chapter and complete the following statements.

1. _____ is the time immediately before, during, and after birth.

2. _____ manifest before age 21 and are lifelong severe chronic disabilities that can be cognitive, physical, or both.

3. _____ manifest before age 18 and have significant subaverage general intellectual functioning and limitations.

4. _____ are a common manifestation of the iris in patients with Down syndrome.

5. _____ is an abnormal increase in mobility within the joint between the first two cervical (neck) vertebrae in patients with Down syndrome.

MULTIPLE CHOICE QUESTIONS

Complete each question by circling the best answer.

1. The causes of intellectual disabilities may be all of the following EXCEPT:
   a. Genetic
   b. Nutritional
   c. Psychological
   d. Psychosocial

2. The most common intellectual disability is:
   a. Mild
   b. Moderate
   c. Severe
   d. Profound

3. All of the following are considered autism spectrum disorders EXCEPT:
   a. Rett syndrome
   b. Childhood disintegrative disorder
   c. Asperger's syndrome
   d. Echolalia

4. All of the following conditions are apparent in patients with Down syndrome EXCEPT:
   a. Congenital heart disease
   b. Thyroid disease
   c. Orthopedic disorders
   d. Diabetes

5. Which of the following conditions would be considered moderate ID?
   a. Learns very few academic skills past the second-grade level
   b. Educable and able to learn some academic skills
   c. Can learn some oral self-care behaviors with supervision
   d. Incapable of total self-care, social skills, or work skills

6. Self-injury behavior has been identified as a stress response to those with an intellectual disability. Self-injury behavior may occur in typically developing children.
   a. Both statements are true.
   b. Both statements are false.
   c. The first statement is true and the second statement is false.
   d. The first statement is false and the second statement is true.

7. Research has discovered certain biochemicals as the cause of autism. One in every 68 children have been diagnosed with some form of autism in the US.
   a. Both statements are true.
   b. Both statements are false.
   c. The first statement is true and the second statement is false.
   d. The first statement is false and the second statement is true.

8. A mild type of autism that exhibits impairment in social settings but no age-appropriate deficits in language, cognitive, or developmental skills is:
   a. Rett syndrome
   b. Classic autism
   c. Asperger syndrome
   d. PDD-NOS

Rudy lives in a group home with five other men who have intellectual disabilities.

Age	27		SCENARIO
Gender	male		**EOE/IOE:**
Height	5'2"		macroglossia
Weight	170 lb		moderate biofilm generalized
B/P	110/75 mm Hg		moderate calculus generalized
Chief Complaint	Lives in a group home, states his toothbrush gets stolen frequently		**Periodontal Findings:** Probe readings 2-5 mm generalized Moderate BOP
Medical History Current Medications			**Radiographic Findings:** stable
Social History			**Dental Findings:** stable

Using the data from this patient, develop a Human Needs Conceptual model for treatment.

Dental Hygiene Diagnosis (unmet human need)	Etiology (due to...)	Signs and Symptoms (evidenced by...)	Patient Goals (expected outcomes)
Protection from Health Risks			
Freedom from Fear and Stress			
Freedom from Pain			
Wholesome Facial Image			
Skin and Mucous Membrane Integrity of the Head and Neck			
Biologically Sound and Functional Dentition			
Conceptualization and Problem Solving			
Responsibility for Oral Health			

61 Orofacial Clefts

SHORT ANSWER QUESTIONS

1. List the three characteristics of orofacial clefts.

_____

_____

_____

_____

_____

2. Briefly discuss reasons why children with orofacial clefts have a high caries risk.

_____

_____

_____

_____

_____

_____

_____

_____

_____

3. Upper lip development occurs during what week of embryological growth?

_____

_____

4. What two processes form the upper lip?

_____

_____

394

FILL IN THE BLANK STATEMENTS

Select the best term from the chapter and complete the following statements.

1. _____ is a cleft of the upper lip, occurs during the fifth week of fetal development.

2. _____ is a cleft of the palate and may occur at any time during development of the palate and at different locations and in different structures of the palate.

3. _____ is a small mandible.

4. _____ is an enlarged tongue.

5. _____ is tongue blockage of ventilation or ventilation obstruction.

6. _____ is the leakage of air into the nasal passages during speech production.

7. _____ is a prosthetic device that seals an opening in the palate while the device is in place.

MULTIPLE CHOICE QUESTIONS

Complete each question by circling the best answer.

1. A removable appliance designed to close a palatal opening is called:
   a. Hawley retainer
   b. Orthopedic appliance
   c. Pediatric denture
   d. Obturator

2. Velopharyngeal dysfunction is a speech disorder that occurs in patients with palatal clefts. Because the the soft palate does not close against the phargyneal wall, air escapes into the nasal cavity producing hypernasal speech.
   a. Both statements are true.
   b. Both statements are false.
   c. The first statement is true and the second statement is false.
   d. The first statement is false and the second statement is true.

3. Orofacial clefts are the second most common birth defect in the US. American Indians, non-Hispanic whites, and Asians are most affected by orofacial clefts.
   a. Both statements are true.
   b. Both statements are false.
   c. The first statement is true and the second statement is false.
   d. The first statement is false and the second statement is true.

4. An incomplete lip cleft only involves soft tissue. An incomplete palatal cleft involves mucosal tissue.
   a. Both statements are true.
   b. Both statements are false.
   c. The first statement is true and the second statement is false.
   d. The first statement is false and the second statement is true.

5. Palatal development occurs during what week of embryological growth?
   a. 12
   b. 13
   c. 14
   d. 15

6. Palatine development progresses from anterior to posterior. Formation of anterior and posterior palate may develop concurrently.
   a. Both statements are true.
   b. Both statements are false.
   c. The first statement is true and the second statement is false.
   d. The first statement is false and the second statement is true.

7. A cleft of the upper lip is called a chelioschisis. A cleft of the palate is called a palatoschisis.
   a. Both statements are true.
   b. Both statements are false.
   c. The first statement is true and the second statement is false.
   d. The first statement is false and the second statement is true.

8. All of the following have a strong correlation non-syndromic orofacial cleft EXCEPT:
   a. Diet
   b. Genetics
   c. Alcohol misuse of mother
   d. Tobacco use of mother

9. Unilateral or bilateral cleft lip is caused by lack of fusion of the median nasal process and the maxillary process. Complete cleft lip is a notch of any depth involving the philtrum; does not invade hard structures or the nostrils.
   a. Both statements are true.
   b. Both statements are false.
   c. The first statement is true and the second statement is false.
   d. The first statement is false and the second statement is true.

10. The interprofessional team members that manage children with orofacial defects include all of the following EXCEPT:
    a. Pediatric dentist
    b. Periodontist
    c. Otolaryngologist
    d. Geneticist

11. What type of cleft lip presents with a notch of any depth that involves the philtrum but not hard tissues or nostrils?
    a. Incomplete unilateral
    b. Incomplete bilateral
    c. Complete unilateral
    d. Complete bilateral

12. What type of cleft palate involves anterior palate, anterior to incisive foramen and palate, extends to posterior to incisive foramen, and includes hard and soft palate?
    a. Complete bilateral
    b. Complete unilateral
    c. Cleft palate only
    d. Submucosal cleft

CASE STUDY: MS. ANYA

Your 20-year-old new patient arrives for a new patient exam. She recently arrived here from Kosovo having been granted legal asylum for humanitarian protection. She has her 2-month-old baby boy in a carrier, and you notice he has a cleft lip and palate. You ask about the baby, and she states that she is concerned about his appearance and his ability to eat properly. What steps do you take to assist this mother? What other professionals do you contact? What education do you provider for her?

_____

_____

_____

_____

_____

_____

_____

_____

_____

_____

_____

396

Chapter **61** Orofacial Clefts

62 Neurologic Disabilities

COMPETENCIES

1. Explain features, symptoms, and considerations for patient management and oral self-care of various dysfunctions of the motor system, including tremors, Parkinson disease, cerebral palsy, multiple sclerosis, amyotrophic lateral sclerosis, and Huntington disease.
2. Explain features, symptoms, and considerations for patient management and oral self-care of various dysfunctions of the central nervous system, including traumatic brain injury and post-traumatic stress disorder, spinal cord injury, seizures, and epilepsy.
3. Explain features, symptoms, and considerations for patient management and oral self-care of various peripheral neuropathies, including facial neuropathy (Bell's palsy) and trigeminal neuralgia.
4. Explain features, symptoms, and considerations for patient management and oral self-care of various disorders of higher cortical function, including dementia and Alzheimer's disease (AD).
5. Explain features, symptoms, and considerations for patient management and oral self-care of cerebrovascular accidents (strokes).
6. Apply knowledge of neurologic disabilities to dental hygiene practice and interprofessional collaboration.

SHORT ANSWER QUESTIONS

1. List and describe the types of cerebral palsy.

_____

_____

_____

_____

2. What are most common oral clinical findings in cerebral palsy patients?

_____

_____

_____

_____

3. Briefly describe Multiple Sclerosis.

_____

_____

_____

_____

4. Briefly describe Amyotrophic Lateral Sclerosis.

_____
_____
_____
_____

5. Briefly describe the three main types of epileptic seizures.

_____
_____
_____
_____
_____
_____
_____
_____

6. List common oral health concerns of patients with MS.

_____
_____
_____
_____
_____
_____
_____
_____

FILL IN THE BLANK STATEMENTS

Select the best term from the chapter and complete the following statements.

1. A mental health condition that occurs following a traumatic event in which someone witnesses or experiences a threat to their physical or emotional well-being is _____.

2. A _____ is a brief disturbance of cerebral function caused by excessive abnormal neuronal discharge.

3. _____ is an increase in muscular movement while _____ is a decrease in muscular movement.

4. Hypersalivation is also known as _____.

5. A brief episode of insufficient blood supply to brain that results in no permanent neurological damage is _____.

6. The inability to initiate voluntary movement is _____.

MULTIPLE CHOICE QUESTIONS

Complete each question by circling the best answer.

1. When communicating with a patient who has Alzheimer's disease, all of the following are suggested communication techniques EXCEPT:
   a. Limit the use of ultrasonic devices
   b. Give patients several choices for care
   c. Explain procedures simply
   d. Speak slowly

2. Risk factors for cerebrovascular accident are all of the following EXCEPT:
   a. Hypertension
   b. Diabetes
   c. High cholesterol
   d. Age 40-65

3. Right-side brain damage characteristics are all of the following EXCEPT:
   a. Paralyzed left side
   b. Perception difficulties
   c. Impulsive behavior
   d. Anxiety

4. Left-side brain damage characteristics are all of the following EXCEPT:
   a. Speech difficulties
   b. Memory difficulties
   c. Unable to use a mirror
   d. Slow behavior

5. What type of seizure results in loss of consciousness?
   a. Myoclonic
   b. Grand mal
   c. Petit mal
   d. TIA

6. What type of seizure results in loss of awareness with no motor activity?
   a. Myoclonic
   b. Grand mal
   c. Petit mal
   d. TIA

7. Sudden unilateral facial paralysis, weakness of the upper and lower facial muscles, drooping eyelids, drooping corner of the mouth, and difficulty eating are the symptoms of:
   a. Bell's Palsy
   b. Epilpesy
   c. Trigeminal neuralgia
   d. Dementia

8. Progressive intellectual decline that eventually leads to deterioration of occupational, social, and interpersonal functions is:
   a. Bell's Palsy
   b. Myasthenia Gravis
   c. Trigeminal neuralgia
   d. Dementia

9. Neuropathy of the trigeminal nerve is:
   a. Bell's Palsy
   b. Multiple Sclerosis
   c. Trigeminal neuralgia
   d. Dementia

10. A stroke is a result of a brief lack of blood supply to the brain. Hemorrhagic stroke is caused by a rupture of a brain vessel that causes leakage of blood into the brain tissue.
    a. Both statements are true.
    b. Both statements are false.
    c. The first statement is true, the second is false.
    d. The first statement is false, the second is true.

11. Death occurs in patients with ALS due to what complication?
    a. Cardiac
    b. Respiratory
    c. CNS degeneration
    d. Stroke

12. All of the following statements are true concerning cerebral palsy EXCEPT:
    a. Non-progressive neuromuscular disorder
    b. Affects ability to control posture and movement
    c. Is caused by muscle and nerve damage
    d. Involves motor areas of the immature brain

13. All of the following are risk factors for cerebral palsy after birth EXCEPT:
    a. Post-term birth
    b. Hypoxic ischemic encephalopathy
    c. Seizures
    d. Low birth weight

14. The type of cerebral palsy that presents with balance, coordination, and depth perception is:
    a. Spastic
    b. Athetoid
    c. Dyskinetic
    d. Ataxic

15. All of the following statements are true concerning multiple sclerosis EXCEPT:
    a. Progressive neurological condition that affects older adults
    b. Myelin sheath destruction
    c. More common in females than males
    d. Symptoms gradually occur over time

Age	62
Gender	female
Height	5'7"
Weight	180 lb
B/P	150/80 mm Hg
Chief Complaint	Difficulty swallowing, sleeping, no dental exam in 2 years
Medical History Current Medications	Diagnosed with ALS 2 years ago Paxil for anxiety Propranolol - beta-adrenergic blocking agent to thin secretions
Social History	Non-drinker, non-smoker Retired nurse

SCENARIO

Patient is confined to a wheelchair, requires assistance with daily activities, has difficulty swallowing

EOE/IOE:
Coated tongue
Moderate biofilm generalized
Slight supragingival calculus generalized

Periodontal Findings:
Generalized bleeding on probing
Probe readings 3-4 posterior, 2-3 anterior
Type I periodontitis
moderate gingival inflammation

Radiographic Findings:
Stable dentition

Dental Findings:
Last dental exam 2 years ago. Last radiographs were 4 years ago. She rates her oral health as fair.

She reports that her caregiver/husband tries to brush her teeth twice a day. No other aids are used.

Caregiver reports that the patient often drools. She must sleep at an incline to prevent aspiration from saliva/mucous

1. What considerations will your operatory setup need?

2. What instructions will the caregiver need?

3. What dietary modifications should be made?

4. Develop a homecare plan for Ms. Perry's caregiver.

_____

_____

_____

_____

5. What treatment will you deliver today?

_____

_____

_____

_____

6. What is your long-term plan for this patient?

_____

_____

_____

_____

63 Professional Development and Job Searching

COMPETENCIES

1. Develop a professional career plan by performing a self-assessment, building a network for professional enhancement and a relationship with a mentor, establishing professional career goals, and creating an action plan.
2. Research employment opportunities to identify a desired dental hygiene position.
3. Prepare for a job application by developing a résumé, cover letter, and list of references; prepare for a job interview by creating a list of personal statements, questions, and other considerations. Communicate effectively in a job interview and follow up appropriately afterward.
4. Prioritize employment factors, including compensation, employment rights and evaluation, the expanding scope of dental hygiene, potential sources of burnout or stress, and professionalism on social media websites while balancing your personal and professional values and needs.
5. Describe the importance of leadership in dental hygiene and lifelong learning for career development.

SHORT ANSWER QUESTIONS

1. List ways to build professional relationships through mentors.

_____

_____

_____

_____

_____

_____

_____

_____

_____

2. List ADHA's opportunities and roles of the dental hygienist.

_____

_____

_____

_____

_____

_____

_____

_____

_____

_____

_____

3. List various compensation methods for dental hygienists.

_____

_____

_____

_____

_____

_____

_____

_____

_____

_____

_____

_____

4. What are sources for career "burnout"?

_____

_____

_____

_____

_____

_____

_____

_____

403

5. List educational advancements in the profession of dental hygiene.

_____

_____

_____

_____

_____

_____

_____

6. List sources for finding dental hygiene employment.

_____

_____

_____

_____

_____

_____

_____

_____

_____

_____

FILL IN THE BLANK STATEMENTS

Select the best term from the chapter and complete the following statements.

1. A _____ is a trusted advisor who can serve as a professional resource and provide guidance for career growth, often through mutual engagement over time.

2. A_____ is developed by creating a list of personal goals that one hopes to attain within his or her career.

3. The _____ is a document that highlights education, experience, skill sets, and achievements that highlight someone's qualifications for a job.

4. An _____, also known as an e-portfolio or digital portfolio, is a digital collection of material that provides evidence supporting your efforts, achievements, and progress gained from education, work, and life experiences.

5. _____ are individuals that provide recommendations for a person who is applying for a job.

404

6. A _____ is an introductory letter, accompanying the résumé, designed to introduce the job candidate to a potential employer.

7. A _____, in which they actually perform the job within the work environment with staff members before being offered the position.

8. _____ to care means that dental hygienists are able to initiate treatment based on their assessment of patients' needs without the specific authorization or presence of a dentist.

MULTIPLE CHOICE QUESTIONS

Complete each question by circling the best answer.

1. A career plan should have short and long-term goals. A career plan should be attainable and have safe boundaries.
   a. Both statements are true.
   b. Both statements are false.
   c. The first statement is true and the second statement is false.
   d. The first statement is false and the second statement is true.

2. Contributing to the dental hygiene body of knowledge is a career path of:
   a. Clinician
   b. Educator
   c. Public health
   d. Research

3. The function of a resume is to:
   a. Give a detailed biography beginning with high school graduation
   b. Highlight skills and accomplishments for desired job
   c. Acquire several references to validate skills
   d. Impress the reader with competent writing skills

4. Dental hygiene career development should begin after graduation. Career development may change along with life's changes.
   a. Both statements are true.
   b. Both statements are false.
   c. The first statement is true and the second statement is false.
   d. The first statement is false and the second statement is true.

5. A high-quality resume should include all of the following EXCEPT:
   a. Professional goals
   b. Summary of responsibilities
   c. Marital status
   d. Professional affiliations

6. The ability of a dental hygienist to initiate patient treatment without specific authorization from a dentist is:
   a. Direct access
   b. Direct supervision
   c. General supervision
   d. Indirect access

7. A digital collection of material that provides support and evidence of a practitioner's achievements, skills, progress, and work is:
   a. E-portfolio
   b. Resume
   c. Letters of recommendation
   d. Performance evaluation

64 Practice Management

COMPETENCIES

1. Describe techniques used for successful practice management.
2. Discuss techniques used for successful patient and record management, including:
   - List the elements of a complete case presentation.
   - Explain the risks of relaxed HIPAA policies and procedure enforcement.
   - Maintain detailed records for each patient.
   - Discuss quality assurance and the record auditing process.
3. List the types of software management systems available as well as their advantages and disadvantages.
4. Discuss time management and scheduling options to create a smooth schedule.
5. Explain economic considerations for a profitable practice, including office overhead, production, and collection.
6. Discuss the marketing of dentistry and dental hygiene, including:
   - List the four P's of marketing.
   - Compare and contrast types of social media used for marketing.
7. Discuss the integral contributions of the dental hygienist to the dental healthcare team.

SHORT ANSWER QUESTIONS

1. List examples of suggested meeting types.

_____

_____

_____

_____

_____

_____

_____

_____

_____

2. What are steps to address conflict resolution?

_____

_____

_____

_____

_____

_____

_____

_____

_____

_____

_____

_____

_____

_____

3. What information should be included in a patient record?

_____

_____

_____

_____

_____

_____

_____

_____

_____

_____

_____

_____

4. What are the elements of a complete case presentation?

_____

_____

_____

_____

_____

_____

_____

_____

_____

_____

_____

_____

FILL IN THE BLANK STATEMENTS

Select the best term from the chapter and complete the following statements.

1. _____ is the organization, administration, and direction of the professional practice in a style that facilitates high-quality patient care, efficient use of time and personnel, reduced stress for staff members and patients, enhanced professional and personal satisfaction for staff, and financial profitability.

2. _____ is a formal summary of the aims and values of a company, organization, or individual.

3. _____ a realistic "why" and "how" about the current state of the practice, point toward the future, and layout strategies that will allow the practice to achieve those goals.

4. _____ is the act of overmanaging by practice leaders.

5. _____ is a style that incorporates team empowerment, shared influence, frequent and constructive communication, and, most importantly, flexibility.

6. _____ is promptly adding treatment entries after any discussion or treatment is performed using clear, concise statements that describe the appointment and signed by the treating clinician.

7. _____ is an online combination of information, such as health histories, medical and dental prescriptions, dental and periodontal charting, medical alerts, radiographs, current and future treatment planning, treatment notes, intra-office communication, oral health education, and other areas that are a part of comprehensive dental care.

8. _____ promotes and sells products or services to the public, and may include market research or advertising, that satisfies the needs and wants of the public through an exchange of paid services – while obtaining and maintaining the patient base needed for a successful practice – all while building a long-term trusting relationship.

9. _____ is online technologies and applications that people use to create and share content that includes insights, experiences, and opinions via social networking.

MULTIPLE CHOICE QUESTIONS

Complete each question by circling the best answer.

1. The main purpose of dental and dental hygiene records is communication. Legal documentation is secondary purpose of the dental and dental hygiene record.
   a. Both statements are true.
   b. Both statements are false.
   c. The first statement is true and the second statement is false.
   d. The first statement is false and the second statement is true.

2. Mixed Marketing includes all of the following EXCEPT:
   a. Promotion
   b. Price
   c. Population
   d. Place

3. Economic considerations within the dental practice include all of the following EXCEPT:
   a. Profit
   b. Social media presence
   c. Production
   d. Patient satisfaction

4. All of the following are necessary quality assurance measures EXCEPT:
   a. Practice-centered standards of care
   b. Routine review of a sample of patient records
   c. Patient care review policies
   d. Means to determine cause of treatment deficiencies

5. All of the following are considered errors to be detected during chart audits EXCEPT:
   a. Educational
   b. Noncritical
   c. Critical
   d. Noneducational

6. All of the following are components of a quality assurance plan EXCEPT:
   a. Practice-centered standards
   b. Ongoing review of patient records
   c. Systems to determine treatment deficits
   d. Chart audits

7. All of the following are types of errors that can discovered during an audit EXCEPT:
   a. Critical
   b. Noncritical
   c. Feedback
   d. Nonessential

65 Telehealth

COMPETENCIES

1. Define key terms related to the use of telehealth technology in oral health care.
2. Compare and contrast the four telehealth delivery modalities.
3. Describe the four common categories of oral health care services delivered via teledentistry.
4. Explain how telehealth technology can be used to decrease barriers to accessing oral health care.
5. Summarize how to adapt the dental hygiene process of care using telehealth technology.

SHORT ANSWER QUESTIONS

1. List the four common categories of oral health care services that can be provided using telehealth technology.

_____

_____

_____

_____

_____

_____

2. List the four telehealth delivery modalities and brief descriptions.

_____

_____

_____

_____

_____

3. List the three categories of telehealth care.

_____

_____

_____

_____

_____

_____

_____

409

4. List technologies that may be used for communications between oral health providers and patients.

_____

_____

_____

_____

_____

FILL IN THE BLANK STATEMENTS

Select the best term from the chapter and complete the following statements.

1. _____ is transmission of patient data through a secure electronic communications system to a health provider who uses the information to evaluate or diagnose a patient's condition and/or update a patient's treatment plan without live interaction.

2. _____ is health and health-related services supported by mobile applications (apps) on smart devices such as cell phones and tablet computers.

3. _____ is personal health and medical data collection from an individual in one location via electronic communication technologies, which is transmitted to a provider or data processing service in a different location for use in care and related supportive care.

4. _____ is live, two-way interaction between a patient, or client, and a health provider using audiovisual telecommunications.

5. _____ is a broad variety of health and health-related services delivered through telecommunications and digital communications technology.

MULTIPLE CHOICE QUESTIONS

Complete each question by circling the best answer.

1. Which of the following allows providers and patients share information directly with each other before or after telehealth appointments?
   a. Remote patient monitoring
   b. Synchronous
   c. Asynchronous
   d. Telehealth

2. What is a type of telehealth in which healthcare providers monitor patients outside the traditional care setting using digital medical devices?
   a. Teleconsultation
   b. Telediagnosis
   c. Mobile Health
   d. Remote Patient Monitoring (RPM)

3. What is a form of teledentistry that screens patients remotely to determine the patient's condition and care needs using a web-based or app-based tool?
   a. Teletriage
   b. Telemonitoring
   c. Teleconsultation
   d. Telediagnosis

4. Health and health-related services that are supported by mobile applications on smart devices are:
   a. Remote Patient Monitoring
   b. mHealth
   c. Synchronous
   d. Asynchronous

5. Oral health providers that perform a remove evaluation and make a diagnosis is:
   a. Telemonitoring
   b. Teleconsultation
   c. Telediagnosis
   d. Telehealth care

6. The electronic transmission of health information to a practitioner who uses the information to evaluate a health condition outside of a live interaction is:
   a. Store and forward
   b. Live video feed
   c. Mobile health
   d. Remote monitoring

CASE STUDY

Your community has hired you to create a program to provide oral health screenings to school-aged children using teledentistry. What technology would you use? What services would you provide? What barriers might you face?

_____

_____

_____

_____

_____

_____

_____

_____

_____

_____

_____

_____

66 Mental Health and Self-Care

COMPETENCIES

1. Discuss the prevalence of anxiety, depression, and increase in mental disorders.
2. Contrast the relationship between stress and stressors.
3. Compare negative short-term and long-term health outcomes to chronic stress, anxiety, and depression.
4. Analyze the occurrence of professional burnout in the dental hygiene profession and describe factors that influence burnout and time off from work.
5. Correlate the importance of early intervention measures to reduce the occurrence of stress related chronic conditions and professional burnout.
6. Identify the impact of the practitioner's mental health as it relates to patient care, as well as the role of the practitioner in addressing the overall well-being of the patient.
7. Integrate self-care and stress management strategies.

SHORT ANSWER QUESTIONS

1. List the four types of stresses.

_____

_____

_____

_____

2. List physical symptoms of stress.

_____

_____

_____

_____

_____

_____

3. List psychological symptoms of stress.

_____

_____

_____

_____

_____

_____

_____

4. List examples of anxiety.

_____

_____

_____

_____

_____

_____

_____

_____

_____

_____

5. List examples of depression.

_____

_____

_____

_____

_____

_____

_____

6. List possible stressors facing dental hygienists.

_____

_____

_____

_____

_____

FILL IN THE BLANK STATEMENTS

Select the best term from the chapter and complete the following statements.

1. _____ is characterized by emotional and physical exhaustion, detachment from work, and feelings of professional loneliness.

2. _____ is regular, sudden attacks of panic or fear.

3. _____ is a persistent fear of being judged or watched by others.

4. _____ is an overall feeling of excessive worry about a variety of topics, resulting in fatigue, inability to focus, sleep disturbance, and feeling on edge.

5. _____ may develop when an individual has experienced a shocking, dangerous, or scary event.

MULTIPLE CHOICE QUESTIONS

Complete each question by circling the best answer.

1. Which type of stress is short-term?
   a. Distress
   b. Acute
   c. Chronic
   d. Eustress

2. Which type of stress is from positive or happy life events?
   a. Distress
   b. Acute
   c. Chronic
   d. Eustress

3. Which type of stress is from negative factors?
   a. Distress
   b. Acute
   c. Chronic
   d. Eustress

4. Which type of stress is long-term?
   a. Distress
   b. Acute
   c. Chronic
   d. Eustress

5. All of the following may prompt dental fear anxiety in a patient EXCEPT:
   a. Smells associated with a dental office
   b. Sounds of dental equipment
   c. No TV's in operatories
   d. Anticipating pain

6. The body's natural response to stress is to:
   a. Secrete endorphins
   b. Run and hide
   c. Panic
   d. Fight or flight

CASE STUDY

Michael, a 10-year seasoned dental hygienist, has been feeling a lot of stress. His office is understaffed to meet the demands of patient care. He is recently separated from his wife and is experiencing symptoms of depression. He feels alone and isolated. What would you recommend to Michael to help him improve his mental state?

_____

_____

_____

_____

_____

_____

_____

_____

_____

_____

_____

_____